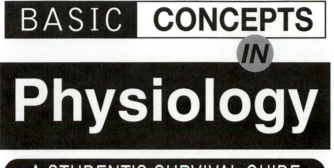

BASIC CONCEPTS IN

Physiology

A STUDENT'S SURVIVAL GUIDE

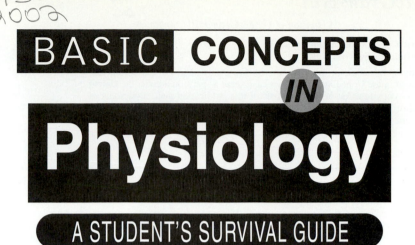

BASIC CONCEPTS *IN*
Physiology

A STUDENT'S SURVIVAL GUIDE

CHARLES SEIDEL, PhD

Professor
Department of Medicine
Department of Molecular Physiology and Biophysics
Baylor College of Medicine
Houston, Texas

McGraw-Hill
Medical Publishing Division

New York   Chicago   San Francisco   Lisbon   London
Madrid   Mexico City   Milan   New Delhi   San Juan
Seoul   Singapore   Sydney   Toronto

McGraw-Hill

A Division of The McGraw·Hill Companies

Notice

Medicine is an ever-changing science. As new research and clinical experience broaden our knowledge, changes in treatment and drug therapy are required. The author and the publisher of this work have checked with sources believed to be reliable in their efforts to provide information that is complete and generally in accord with the standards accepted at the time of publication. However, in view of the possibility of human error or changes in medical sciences, neither the author nor the publisher nor any other party who has been involved in the preparation or publication of this work warrants that the information contained herein is in every respect accurate or complete, and they disclaim all responsibility for any errors or omissions or for the results obtained from use of the information contained in this work. Readers are encouraged to confirm the information contained herein with other sources. For example and in particular, readers are advised to check the product information sheet included in the package of each drug they plan to administer to be certain that the information contained in this work is accurate and that changes have not been made in the recommended dose or in the contraindications for administration. This recommendation is of particular importance in connection with new or infrequently used drugs.

This book was set in Times Roman by Pine Tree Composition, Inc.
The editors were Janet Foltin, Harriet Lebowitz, and Karen Davis.
The production supervisor was Lisa Mendez.
The cover designer was Mary McDonnell.
The index was prepared by Marilyn Rowland.
Artwork was done by Charles Seidel.
R. R. Donnelley, Crawfordsville, was printer and binder.

This book is printed on acid-free paper.

Library of Congress Cataloging-in-Publication Data

Seidel, Charles L.
    Basic concepts in physiology : a student's survival guide / Charles Seidel.—1st ed.
      p. ; cm.
    Includes index.
    ISBN 0-07-135656-8 (alk. paper)
    1. Human physiology.   I. Title.
    [DNLM: 1. Physiological Processes. QT 104 S4565b 2001]
  QP34.5 .S423 2001
  612—dc21

                            2001032984

INTERNATIONAL EDITION ISBN 0-07-115065-X

Copyright © 2002. Exclusive rights by The McGraw-Hill Companies, Inc., for manufacture and export. This book cannot be reexported from the country to which it is consigned by McGraw-Hill. The International Edition is not available in North America.

· C O N T E N T S ·

v

CHAPTER 3   CARDIOVASCULAR SYSTEM   35

CHAPTER 4   RENAL PHYSIOLOGY   74

CHAPTER 5   RESPIRATORY PHYSIOLOGY   102

CHAPTER 6   GASTROINTESTINAL PHYSIOLOGY   128

CHAPTER 7   ENDOCRINE PHYSIOLOGY 161

CHAPTER 8   TEMPERATURE REGULATION   **205**

· P R E F A C E ·

The depth of physiological knowledge has increased tremendously since the application of molecular biological and genetic techniques. However, this depth is overwhelming if the basic physiological concepts are not first understood. It is the goal of this book to help you acquire this basic understanding so that the additional details are more fully appreciated. Although this book covers normal human physiology, clinical examples are included periodically to illustrate how changes in the normal can lead to pathology.

The book is written for students interested in determining whether or not they have mastered the basic concepts in physiology. But the beginning student should find it useful either as a supplement to an in-depth textbook or as a primary source in an introductory human physiology course.

To help you study efficiently, the book is divided into short sections each beginning with the key points of the section highlighted in a box. If the information in the box is familiar and you can expand on the items listed, then skip to the next box. However, if the information is unfamiliar, read the text that follows. In this way you can quickly determine which areas need additional study.

No book can be written without the help of others. First, I want to thank Susan Hamilton and Mark Entman for relieving me of some of my departmental duties, which enabled me to have time to write. I am indebted to my colleagues Ashok Balasubramanyam, Mary Hamra, and Mike Reid for reading various sections. Their comments and encouragement were greatly appreciated. But I take full responsibility for not always following their suggestions. I also appreciate the patience of the editors Janet Foltin and Harriet Lebowitz as they accommodated their schedule to mine. Finally, this book would not exist had not my wife, Mary, given up many weekends to my slow methodical writing.

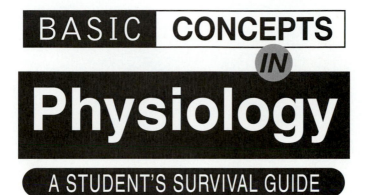

BASIC CONCEPTS IN Physiology

A STUDENT'S SURVIVAL GUIDE

HOMEOSTASIS

·

DEFINITION OF PHYSIOLOGY

> • Physiology is the study of how things work.

Knowing the names of components and how they are assembled into a working system is important so that you can talk about them. For example, to talk about how an automobile engine works and how to fix it, you need a vocabulary describing the components of the engine. You need to be able to identify a carburetor, an air filter, a spark plug, an oxygen sensor, a camshaft and so on. You also need to know their location on the engine in case they are missing or inappropriately positioned. Naming the component parts of the human body is the purview of histology and gross anatomy.

You cannot be a competent mechanic, however, if you do not know what the component parts do and how they interact with one another. Understanding how the parts of the human body work together is the purview of physiology.

BASIC PRINCIPLE OF PHYSIOLOGY

> • Homeostasis is the basic principle of physiology.
> • Homeostasis is the maintenance of a constant environment.

Homeostasis is the maintenance of a constant environment. What enables us to live, work, and learn under changing conditions of temperature and humidity is to be able to surround ourselves with a hospitable environment generated by systems that heat, cool, and dehumidify the air. Whether in buildings, homes or

1

automobiles, these systems are in constant struggle with the external environment. They are trying to maintain a hospitable internal environment against an inhospitable external environment. The body does the same thing. For the body, the external environment may be the outside physical world or the environment surrounding individual cells or organs.

To understand physiology is to understand how the body's homeostatic systems work. A key to learning physiology is to organize the information into homeostatic systems.

COMPONENTS OF A HOMEOSTATIC SYSTEM

> • Regulated variable is a variable to be kept constant.
> • Set point is the desired value for the regulated variable.
> • Sensors assess current status of the regulated variable.
> • Feedback controller compares current conditions with the set point.
> • Effector brings current status of regulated variable into line with the set point.

Any homeostatic system has five common components (see Figure 1–1). The first component is the thing that needs to be kept constant. In a house this may be the temperature. This is called the *regulated variable*. Temperature, blood pressure, and the blood content of glucose, oxygen, and potassium ions are examples of regulated variables in the body. The body wants these variables to stay at a certain level. Not everything is a regulated variable. Heart rate, cardiac output, vascular resistance, urine output, and breathing rate are not regulated variables. These things may change, but they usually change in order to keep the regulated variable constant. If you remember what things are regulated variables, you will be a long way toward understanding the details of the homeostatic responses of the body. Once you know the regulated variable, in many cases you will be able to identify intuitively how the body might keep it constant.

Another aspect of a homeostatic system is that it must "know" what is normal. "Normal" is where the regulated variable should be. This normal condition is called the *set point*. For example, if the thermostat in your house is set at 76°F, this temperature is the set point that the air conditioning system tries to maintain. For every regulated variable there is a set point. Therefore, the body has set points for temperature, blood pressure, and the blood content of oxygen, glucose, and potassium. You need to know the value of these set points so that you will recognize if something is wrong. If my wife and I don't agree on the set point for the thermostat, I might interpret a temperature greater than 76 as a sign that the air conditioner is broken. However, this may be the set point that my wife has selected. Some diseases involve changes in the body's set point. You shiver when

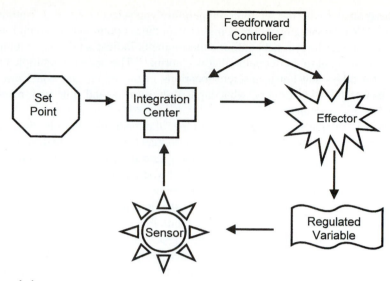

Figure 1–1
A standard homeostatic system consists of five elements: set point, sensor, integration center, effector, and regulated variable. Most homeostatic systems are designed to keep the regulated variable equal to the set point.

you have a fever because the temperature set point of your body has been increased. Your body tries to generate heat to raise its temperature by contracting the skeletal muscles. High blood pressure (hypertension) can be maintained because the set point for blood pressure is increased and the body initiates responses to maintain the blood pressure at this elevated level. So, it is important to know the normal set point and to realize that the set point can be changed as part of a disease process. An illness can result from the use of normal body responses to maintain an abnormal set point.

The third component of a homeostatic system is some mechanism by which the body can "know" the current conditions. There has to be a *sensor* that monitors the internal environment. For example, the thermostat senses the air temperature in your house. For every regulated variable there has to be a sensor. Therefore, the body has sensors for temperature, blood pressure, blood osmolarity, and the blood content of glucose, oxygen, and potassium, to name a few. Part of the study of physiology is the study of these sensors. You will learn where they are located, how they sense, the nature of their response to changes in the regulated variable, and where they send their information.

The information from the sensor about the current value of the regulated variable is useless if there is no way to compare the signals coming from the sensor with the set point. There has to be a *feedback controller* or *integrating center*. The thermostat in your house compares the current air temperature as sensed by the thermometer with the set point temperature you selected. If the thermometer indicates that the air temperature is higher than the set point, the air conditioning will turn on. It will remain on until the thermometer indicates that the air temperature is now equal to the set point, that is, "normal." The body has multiple feedback controllers that are in discrete locations in the brain. You will learn the locations of these controllers, what input they receive, and how they respond under specific circumstances.

In the example of a home air conditioner, the feedback controller had a way to produce change—to alter the internal environment so that the actual air temperature became equal to the set point. A homeostatic system must have an *effector*, that is, some way to produce a change. The home air conditioner is the effector that cools the air and blows the cooled air around inside the house in order to return the temperature to the set point. The body also has effectors and you will be spending a lot of your time understanding them. For example, to maintain temperature, the body uses skin blood flow, sweat production, and skeletal muscle contraction as effectors to either lower or increase body temperature to keep it at the set point. To maintain blood pressure the body alters the pumping action of the heart through changes in its rate of beating and its output per beat (stroke volume), the resistance of the vasculature to blood flow, and the volume of blood.

CHARACTERISTICS OF HOMEOSTASIS

- Effectors may have opposing actions.
- Negative feedback is the process that prevents change.
- Positive feedback is the process that perpetuates change.
- Feedforward control is outside stimuli that alter the normal feedback response.

Returning again to the example of a home air conditioner, notice that if the temperature of the house falls below the set point, nothing happens. The air conditioning system only prevents the house temperature from rising above the set point. It does nothing to actively warm the house if the temperature falls below the set point. For example, the furnace does not turn on if the temperature falls below a set point of 76°F. Few if any systems in the body work this way. The great majority of systems are constructed so that a corrective response is initiated if conditions move above or below the set point. This means that the effectors have opposite or competing actions.

This can be seen at two levels. At the level of a given regulated variable, such as temperature, some effectors raise temperature and some decrease temperature. They compete with or oppose each other to keep temperature constant. Around each regulated variable there is a constellation of effectors each exerting an action. These effects balance, keeping the temperature constant. A steady state is established because of these competing actions. On a more global scale, conflicts can develop between effectors interacting to maintain different regulated variables. For example, when you run in a hot, humid environment, there is a conflict between the effectors that are trying to maintain body temperature and those that are trying to maintain blood pressure. As your body temperature rises, more blood is directed to your skin to try to lower body temperature. However, this means that there is less blood to supply exercising muscle. Something has to give. In this example, temperature wins. The body does not want to "cook" the brain, so skeletal muscle blood flow is sacrificed to preserve appropriate temperature. So there is a hierarchy to the regulated variables. This is a very important point, which, if forgotten, can lead to confusion.

A term used to describe the process by which a regulated variable is maintained constant is *negative feedback*. Discrepancies between the set point and the regulated variable set into motion processes that attempt to return the regulated variable to the set point. If blood pressure rises, actions are taken to lower blood pressure. The initial response elicits an opposite response. This is a closed system that is self-correcting. Sometimes, however, there are situations where the initial response produces further change in the same direction. This is self-perpetuating and is called *positive feedback*. Changes in ion flux that initiate an action potential, blood coagulation, and ovulation are examples of positive feedback systems. There are not many such systems in the body because they do not keep things constant.

There are also situations when information comes from outside the negative feedback loop, information not detected by the sensor, that initiates change. This information usually comes from the brain as it responds to input from sensors outside the feedback loop. A good example is the response to a frightening experience. Your heart rate, blood pressure, and breathing rate increase because of central stimulation, not because of some change in a regulated variable. This type of input is called *feedforward control*. The intrinsic negative feedback systems would antagonize feedforward control unless the set point is changed.

COMMUNICATION IS AN ESSENTIAL ELEMENT OF A HOMEOSTATIC SYSTEM

- Two languages of communication are chemical and electrical.
- Characteristics of communication are distance, speed, distribution.

The sensor has to communicate with the feedback controller and the feedback controller has to communicate with the effector. There are essentially two languages of communication. One is chemical and the other is electrical. These will be developed in later chapters.

Communication has several characteristics: (1) distance: short vs. long; (2) speed: fast vs. slow; and (3) distribution: focused vs. diffuse. Communication occurs over distances as short as the environment surrounding a single cell. Cells can stimulate themselves, called *autocrine stimulation*, or their neighbor, called *paracrine stimulation* through the release of chemical agents. Communication can also occur over long distances, such as a nerve cell located in the spinal cord sending a process out to the end of the finger to stimulate a muscle cell. Communication can be fast, again like nerve stimulation of a muscle cell or the electrical communication between cells during the heartbeat. And it can be slow. Slow communication occurs when the transmission of the chemical is determined by its distribution in the blood. The response to a hormone is intrinsically slower than that to nerve stimulation. Finally, communication can be very focused, such as the activation of single muscle cells in the eye in order to focus on an object. And it can be diffuse, such as when epinephrine, released from the adrenal medulla when blood pressure falls, acts on the heart and the vasculature throughout the whole body.

CELL PHYSIOLOGY

·

MOVEMENT OF MOLECULES ACROSS CELL MEMBRANES

General Properties

- Lipid composition of the cell membrane limits transmembrane movement of molecules.
- The cell membrane is semipermeable because channel and carrier molecules enable some molecules to cross the membrane.
- Channels are proteins that form holes in the cell membrane enabling specific water-soluble molecules to pass in and out of the cell.
- Carriers are proteins that physically move specific molecules across the cell membrane.

The mammalian cell membrane is composed of two layers of lipids (fat) in which protein molecules are embedded. The water-loving (hydrophilic) ends of the lipids face either the exterior or interior of the cell while the water-hating (hydrophobic) ends of the lipid face the interior of the membrane. The protein molecules embedded in this sea of lipids may be large enough to completely span the thickness of the membrane, or they may be confined to one side or the other of the membrane. These proteins form structures such as chemical receptors, attachment points to the extracellular matrix, and transport molecules.

Because of the lipid composition and molecular organization of the cell membrane many molecules cannot cross without assistance. The cell membrane is therefore, said to be selectively permeable or *semipermeable.* Some of the proteins in the cell membrane form structures that permit transmembrane movement of such molecules. There are two ways that the cell gets molecules through the

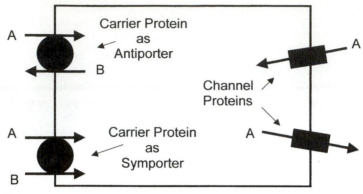

Figure 2–1
Nonlipid-soluble molecules move across cell membranes either through channels or by carrier proteins.

lipid-rich membrane (see Figure 2–1). One way is for proteins to form water-filled *channels* while the other is for the proteins to actually carry the molecule through the membrane. Movement of molecules by *carrier proteins* is also called *facilitated transport.* A significant correlate of the presence of channel and carrier proteins is that the channels and carriers become points of control by which the movement of molecules into and out of the cell is regulated. Many hormones, neurotransmitters, and pharmaceutical agents alter the normal state of channel or carrier proteins as part of their mechanism of action.

Channel Proteins

- Channel proteins are molecules that form water-filled holes through the cell membrane.
- Molecules move through channels by diffusion down concentration gradients.
- Opening and closing (conductance) of channels is controlled.
- Movement through channels cannot be saturated.

The movement of molecules, primarily ions, through channels is dependent on two factors (see Figure 2–1). The first is the *conductance* of the channel, that is, whether or not the channel is open. The second is the *concentration gradient* of the molecule across the cell membrane. Since the channel provides only a path through the membrane for the molecule to follow, net movement through a channel always occurs down a concentration gradient. Movement is due to passive diffusion of the molecule. As long as the channel is open, the rate of movement of a molecule through the channel will increase in proportion to the concentration gradient. This means that the movement of molecules through a channel does not reach a maximum as the concentration increases. In other words, movement through channels is not *saturated*. This is a characteristic that distinguishes movement through channels from movement by carriers. Channels can be very specific in that they allow the passage of a single type of molecule, eg, sodium ions. Alternatively, they can be less selective, permitting the passage of classes of molecules, eg, cations.

Carrier Proteins

- Carrier proteins interact with the molecule being moved and facilitate its movement through the membrane.
- Carriers can become saturated.
- Movement of molecules by carriers can be passive and dependent upon concentration gradients or active and dependent upon energy from ATP.
- Carriers may or may not move multiple molecules simultaneously.
- A carrier that moves a single molecule is called a uniporter.
- A carrier that moves two molecules simultaneously in the same direction (co-transport) is called a symporter.
- A carrier that moves two molecules simultaneously in opposite directions (counter-transport) is called an antiporter.
- In secondary active transport, the active transport of molecules by one carrier drives the passive movement of molecules by another carrier protein.

The movement of molecules by carrier proteins has characteristics that are different in several ways from movement through channels (see Figure 2–1). Because the carrier protein interacts with the molecule to be "carried" and there are a finite number of carrier molecules in the cell membrane, there are a maximum number of molecules that can be carried. As the concentration of molecules to be carried increases, more and more of the carriers become occupied and net movement reaches a maximum. At this point it is said that the carrier has become saturated. *Saturation* is a characteristic of all carrier-mediated movement. Because the carrier protein interacts with the molecule to be carried, the second characteristic of carrier molecules is that they physically facilitate the movement of molecules through the membrane. Carrier proteins enable *facilitated transport* of molecules.

Carrier-mediated facilitated transport is of two types. One type is passive where movement is produced by a concentration gradient for one of the molecules to be transported. The second type is active where the carrier protein is an enzyme that utilizes the energy from adenosine triphosphate (ATP) to move molecules against a concentration gradient. Another characteristic of carrier proteins is that they can couple the movement of multiple molecules. When a carrier protein couples the movement of two or more molecules in the same direction, then it is called a *symporter* and the molecules are said to be *co-transported*. If the carrier protein couples the movement of molecules in opposite directions, then it is called an *antiporter* and the molecules are said to be *counter-transported*. If the carrier molecule moves only a single molecule in a particular direction then it is called a *uniporter.*

The molecules moved by one carrier protein can be linked to the movement of molecules by another carrier protein (see Figure 2–1). An example is the relationship between the carrier proteins Na^+-K^+-ATPase and Na^+-glucose symporter in renal epithelial cells. The active transport of Na^+ out of the cell by the Na^+-K^+-ATPase maintains a low intracellular Na^+ concentration. The movement of Na into the cell down this concentration gradient is mediated by a symporter that also brings glucose into the cell against a concentration gradient. In this way, the potential energy stored in the Na concentration gradient is used to move another molecule (glucose) across the cell membrane against a concentration gradient. The movement of glucose is said to occur by a process called *secondary active transport* because the consumption of ATP (by the Na-K-ATPase) is not directly utilized in moving glucose against a concentration gradient.

Osmosis and Osmotic Pressure (see Figure 2–2)

- Osmosis is the movement of water down its concentration gradient.
- Osmosis is determined by the number of impermeable molecules.
- Osmotic pressure is the force drawing water down its concentration gradient.

In contrast to other molecules, water molecules move freely across the membranes of most cells in the body. Water movement occurs by passive diffusion and therefore, is determined by the water concentration gradient. Like other molecules, water molecules move from a high to a low concentration. If you have two containers of equal volume, one containing only water (A in Figure 2–2) and the other containing a mixture of water and an impermeable salt (B in Figure 2–2), the container with the water–salt mixture will have fewer water molecules in it than the container with pure water. Water molecules and salt molecules both occupy space in the volume and so the more of one type of molecule the less there can be of the other in a given volume. If a membrane separates the two volumes and allows water to pass but not salt, water will leave the container of pure water (A) and enter the container with the mixture (B) because of the difference in water concentration. Water is drawn from one container to the other because of the unequal concentration of water. Water movement down its concentration

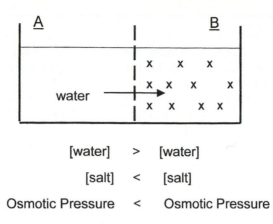

$$[water] \quad > \quad [water]$$

$$[salt] \quad < \quad [salt]$$

$$Osmotic\ Pressure \quad < \quad Osmotic\ Pressure$$

Figure 2–2
Osmosis is the movement of water from a high concentration to a low concentration. In this illustration, two compartments (A and B) are separated by a semipermeable membrane (broken vertical line). The water concentration in compartment A is greater than the concentration in compartment B because of the presence of salt (X) in B. Therefore, water will move down its concentration gradient from A to B. The force needed to prevent this water movement is called osmotic pressure.

gradient is called *osmosis*. Because of osmosis, the volume of the water–salt mixture will increase. To prevent this and keep the two volumes equal, one has to force the water back through the membrane into the chamber of pure water. Pushing down on the liquid in the water–salt container can do this. The amount one would have to push, that is, the amount of pressure one would have to apply to prevent water movement, is called the *osmotic pressure*. Osmotic pressure can also be viewed as the force drawing water molecules from one container to the other. The water–salt solution is exerting an osmotic pressure on the water molecules in the container of pure water. The more salt in the water–salt mixture, that is, the more impermeable particles present, the greater its osmotic pressure because less water is in the mixture and the greater is the difference in water concentration between the two containers.

Tonicity

- The tonicity of a solution refers to the effect of the solution on cell volume.
- A hypertonic extracellular solution is one in which the water concentration is less outside the cell than inside; water leaves the cell; cell volume decreases.

(continued)

(*continued*)
- An isotonic extracellular solution is one in which the water concentration is the same inside and outside the cell; no water movement; cell volume does not change.
- A hypotonic solution is one in which the water concentration is greater outside than inside the cell; water enters the cell; cell volume increases.
- An isosmotic solution may not be an isotonic solution if the particles are permeable to the cell membrane.

Cells in the body shrink or swell in response to the osmotic pressure of the solution surrounding them. Cells are not bags of pure water but contain a variety of molecules in solution, some of which can move across the cell membrane and some of which cannot. The solution surrounding the cells of the body, the *extracellular fluid*, also contains a variety of molecules, some of which can move across the cell membrane and some of which cannot. Because there are molecules both inside and outside the cell that cannot cross the cell membrane, each solution exerts an osmotic pressure. Cells will not change volume when the osmotic pressure exerted by the solution inside the cell *(intracellular fluid)* equals the osmotic pressure exerted by the extracellular fluid. This is an *isotonic* situation because no change in cell volume occurs. The tonicity of the extracellular fluid is a regulated variable maintained by a homeostatic process that makes use of the sensory system to alter the drive for salt and water consumption and the kidneys to regulate the elimination of salt and water.

If the intracellular fluid and extracellular fluid osmotic pressures are not equal, water will move across the cell membrane until the pressures are equal, which will cause the cell volume to either increase or decrease. If the water concentration of the extracellular fluid is less than the intracellular fluid, the cell volume decreases and the extracellular fluid is said to be *hypertonic*. Looking at this in another way, the hypertonic extracellular fluid contains more particles that are unable to cross the cell membrane than does the intracellular fluid. Or, the extracellular fluid contains more osmotically active particles than the intracellular fluid. Therefore, the extracellular fluid has a greater osmotic pressure and water is drawn from the cell. If the water concentration of the extracellular fluid bathing the cell is greater than the intracellular fluid, the cell volume increases and the extracellular fluid is said to be *hypotonic*. The hypotonic extracellular fluid contains fewer molecules that cannot cross the cell membrane than does the intracellular fluid and so is less osmotically active. It, therefore, exerts a lower osmotic pressure than the intracellular fluid and so water is drawn into the cell. If no change in cell volume occurs, then the extracellular fluid is *isotonic*. An isotonic solution contains the same number of molecules that cannot cross the cell membrane as the intracellular fluid.

The difference between an *isosmotic* and an isotonic solution further emphasizes the importance of the permeability properties of the molecules in solution. A solution that contains the same number of particles as are contained within the cell is called an *isosmotic* solution. To determine if this solution is also isotonic, one needs to determine what happens to cell volume when cells are placed in the solution. If the particles are impermeable then there will be no volume change and the isosmotic solution will be isotonic. However, if the particles are permeable they will enter the cell, water will follow, and the cell volume will increase. In this case, the isosmotic solution is really hypotonic. So, again, both the number and permeability of the particles are important.

ELECTRICAL PROPERTIES OF THE CELL
Membrane Potential

- The membrane potential results from charge separation between inside and outside the cell due to the semipermeable nature of the membrane.
- Normally the inside of the cell is negative relative to outside.
- The value of the membrane potential is determined by the ion with greatest permeability.
- The Nernst equation predicts the equilibrium potential.

The membrane of all cells of the body exhibits a small difference in electrical charge between the inside and outside of the cell called the *membrane potential*. This electrical difference is very small, just a few thousandths of a volt (40–90 mV). By convention the membrane potential is measured relative to the outside of the cell and because of this convention is recorded as a negative potential (eg, −80 mV). The membrane potential is the result of differences in membrane permeability of various charged molecules. How a membrane potential comes about and why it is negative is diagramed in Figure 2–3. In Cell A, K ions are in higher concentration inside the cell than outside and can leave the cell through K^+ channels. Molecule P^-, a large negatively charged protein, is also at a higher concentration inside the cell, but it cannot cross the cell membrane. As the positively charged K ion leaves the cell, the negatively charged P is left behind making the inside of the cell negative compared to the outside. The more K ions that leave the cell, the greater will be the charge difference between the inside and outside of the cell. So, it is the difference in permeability properties between K^+ and P^- that permits charge to be separated and a membrane potential established.

However, as the inside of the cell becomes more negative, the negative charge attracts K ions back into the cell. At some point, the movement of K^+ into the cell (due to an electrical gradient) will balance the movement of K^+ out of the cell (due to a concentration gradient). The membrane potential when this balance

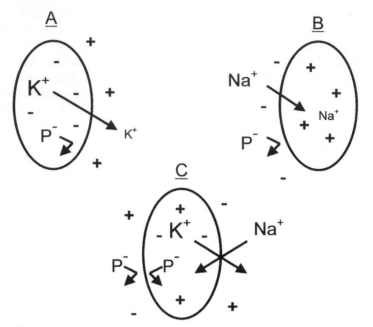

Figure 2–3

Three different cells (A, B, and C) are shown, which contain different amounts of K^+, Na^+, and impermeable protein (P^-). Cell A illustrates how the movement of K^+ out of the cell causes the inside of the cell to become negative. Cell B illustrates how the movement of Na^+ into the cell causes the inside of the cell to become positive. Cell C combines these two effects. For cell C, the membrane potential depends upon the relative permeabilities of K^+ and Na^+ ions.

is achieved is called the *equilibrium potential*. The magnitude of the equilibrium potential is directly related to the concentration difference of the molecule between inside and outside the cell.

Examination of Cell B in Figure 2–3 illustrates that a situation exists that is opposite to that seen in cell A. Because Na ions can enter the cell but P ions cannot, as Na^+ moves into the cell, the outside of the cell becomes negatively charged and the inside becomes positively charged. Again, as the negative charge increases outside the cell, there will be an electrical gradient enhancing the movement of Na^+ out of the cell. There will be an equilibrium potential for Na^+ too, just like for K^+, but it will be in the opposite direction (positive inside to negative outside).

Cell C illustrates the situation when both conditions are combined. Movement of K^+ out of the cell would make the inside negative while Na^+ movement into the cell would make the inside positive. So, which one wins? The final membrane potential will depend upon which ion, Na^+ or K^+, is more permeable. If K^+

is more permeable, then the membrane potential will be closer to the K^+ equilibrium potential. If Na^+ is more permeable, then it will be closer to the Na^+ equilibrium potential. It can also be seen that the membrane potential can be changed from negative inside (K^+ more permeable) to positive inside (Na^+ more permeable) just by adjusting the permeability of K and Na ions. This is exactly what the cell does. Under resting conditions, the permeability of the cell membrane to K^+ is much greater than it is to Na ions. Therefore, the membrane potential is close to the K^+ equilibrium potential. This is why the membrane potential is inside negative. However, under some circumstances (see Action Potential below) the permeabilities of Na^+ and K^+ are changed and the membrane potential moves toward the Na^+ equilibrium potential.

In the late 1800s, Walther Nernst mathematically described the relationship between the equilibrium potential and the concentration gradient of an ion across the cell membrane. This equation, the *Nernst equation* states that for a positive ion I, the equilibrium potential equals the product of a constant K and the log of the ratio of outside and inside concentrations of I.

$$E_I = K \log [I]_o / [I]_I$$

The constant K (RT/ZF) is made up of the gas constant R, the absolute temperature T, the valance Z, and the Faraday constant F. For a monovalent cation at 37°C K equals 61. Each ion would have its own equilibrium potential and the magnitude of the potential would depend on the concentration gradient across the membrane. Once again looking at cell C, the Nernst equation predicts that the equilibrium potential for K^+ would be negative while that for Na^+ would be positive since K_o is less than K_i and Na_o is greater than Na_i. Assuming that K equals 61 (it does) pick some numbers for K^+ and Na^+ and see what concentrations are needed for each to generate a K^+ equilibrium potential of -90 mV and a Na^+ equilibrium potential of $+67$ mV.

Alterations in the Membrane Potential

- Changes in ion conductance alter the membrane potential.
- Hyperpolarization is an increase in membrane potential; inside of the cell becomes more negative; membrane potential moves away from zero.
- Depolarization is a decrease in membrane potential; inside of the cell becomes more positive; membrane potential moves towards zero.

One of the ways that charged substances like K^+ and Na^+ move across the cell membrane is through channels (see preceding discussion). The ability of an ion to move across the membrane through a channel is controlled by the number of channels that are open at any time and the duration that any channel is open. If either of these increase, the ion will move more easily through the membrane. Another term used to describe the ease with which ions move through channels, is *conductance*, sometimes abbreviated "g." K^+ dominates the membrane potential because K^+ conductance (g_K) is greater than Na^+ conductance (g_{Na}). By changing the conductance of one or more ions, the membrane potential can be made to undergo large, rapid and reversible changes in value.

In example C above, if g_K increases, more K^+ will leave the cell and this will make the inside of the cell more negative. The membrane potential will increase and the cell will become *hyperpolarized*. If g_{Na} increases, the inside of the cell will become more positive. The membrane potential will decrease and the cell will become *depolarized*.

In all cells of the body, the intracellular K ion concentration is greater than the extracellular concentration and the extracellular Na ion concentration is greater than the intracellular concentration. These concentration gradients are established and maintained by the counter-transporter (antiporter) Na-K-ATPase. The Na-K-ATPase moves two K ions into the cell and three Na ions out of the cell for each ATP consumed. This means that the Na-K-ATPase also helps make the inside of the cell negative, however, the major determinant of the membrane potential is the passive movement of K^+ out of the cell down its concentration gradient.

Action Potential (see Figure 2–4)

- The action potential is a large, rapid, reversible decrease in membrane potential.
- The action potential usually occurs because of sequential increases in the conductance of Na, Ca, and K ions.
- Threshold is the magnitude of membrane potential that induces an increase in Na^+ conductance.
- Voltage gated channels open and close in response to the membrane potential.
- The refractory period is the period during which the cell is resistant to a second action potential.
- Repolarization is the return of the membrane potential to its original value after the action potential due to an increase in K^+ permeability.
- Excitable cells have action potentials; inexcitable cells do not.

An *action potential* is a large, rapid, and reversible decrease in the cell's membrane potential (depolarizaton). It may last between 2 to 200 thousandths of a second (msec) depending upon the cell type. At the peak of the action potential,

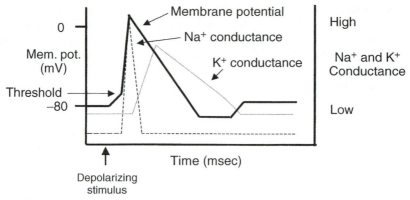

Figure 2–4
Changes in Na⁺ and K⁺ conductance cause the membrane potential to change and generate an action potential. Notice that once the membrane is depolarized above threshold, there is a rapid but transient increase in Na⁺ conductance that produces the depolarizing upstroke of the action potential. Depolarization causes the membrane potential to go towards zero, that is, become smaller. Shortly after this, the K⁺ conductance increases, repolarizing or increasing the membrane potential.

the membrane potential may be close to zero or even inside positive. Because the membrane potential is decreasing during an action potential, it must be the result of a large, rapid, and reversible increase in movement of positive charge into the cell (or negative charge out of the cell). This can be seen from Figure 2–3C. If there were a large influx of Na ions, then the membrane potential would decrease. This influx of positive charge results from a spontaneous, reversible change in the membrane conductance of one or more ions. Generally, the ion channels involved are the Na⁺ and Ca⁺⁺ channels. This makes sense when one remembers that there is a large concentration gradient for these ions from outside to inside the cell. Not all cells can generate an action potential. Those that can are called *excitable cells,* while those that cannot are called *inexcitable cells.* What distinguishes an excitable from an inexcitable cell is the ability of an excitable cell to undergo this spontaneous change in ionic conductance required to generate the action potential.

Before an excitable cell can generate an action potential, its membrane potential must first decrease below a specific value called the *threshold potential.* How this initiating decrease in membrane potential occurs is discussed later. In response to the lower value of the membrane potential, an ion channel (Na and/or Ca) becomes activated and increases its conductance producing a rapid fall in potential characteristic of the action potential (see Figure 2–4). However, the increase in channel conductance is short lived because the falling membrane potential also initiates an inactivation process. The inactivation process returns the conductance of the channel to its original level. For this process to be repeated, the membrane potential must be returned to its resting value, that is, repolarized. If this does not occur, the channels responsible for depolarization (eg, Na, Ca) will not be able to be activated and the production of action potentials will be prevented.

To *repolarize* the membrane, either positive charge must leave the cell or negative charge must enter (see Figure 2–3C). In general, repolarization is the result of an increase in K^+ conductance enabling increased K^+ efflux. Again, this makes sense since the transmembrane concentration gradient for K^+ favors its movement out of the cell. Just as the channels responsible for depolarization are sensitive to the magnitude of the membrane potential, the channels involved with repolarization are also. Depolarization activates these channels (eg, K) but only after a delay, so the increase in their conductance does not occur simultaneously with the increased conductance of channels (eg, Na) responsible for the depolarizing phase of the action potential. Because of the delay in activation, these channels are also called *delayed rectifiers*. The number of ion channels activated, the duration that they remain activated, and the magnitude of the delay before activation determine the shape and magnitude of an action potential in any excitable cell. The shapes of action potentials in skeletal and cardiac muscle cells are dramatically different because the Na, Ca, and K channels in these two cell types have very different properties.

The exact mechanism by which the channel protein senses the value of the membrane potential is not completely known at this time, but genetic studies have identified specific regions of the channel protein or specific conformations of the protein that are involved in activation and inactivation. Since these channel proteins respond to voltage changes they are called *voltage-gated channels*. This is in contrast to channels sensitive to chemical agents that will be described later.

Because channel inactivation occurs spontaneously over a time period characteristic of the channel, a time-dependent modification of the channel must have been set into motion by the activating depolarization. The mechanism of this process is not known. However, if after an action potential the membrane potential is not returned to its original value (ie, repolarized) the inactivation is not removed, the channel cannot be opened again (activated), and another action potential is prevented. During the time course of a normal action potential, there is a period of time during which another action potential cannot be initiated because the inactivation has not been removed from the channels. This is called the *refractory period*.

The depolarization that decreases the membrane potential to threshold may result from an electrical, chemical, or mechanical stimulus. However, in some cells no external stimulus is needed. For example, specialized cells in a region of the right atrium of the heart called the sinoatrial node rhythmically increase g_{Na} and g_{Ca}. These conductance changes enable Na and Ca ions to move into the cell, producing depolarization and initiating an action potential. This action potential propagates through the heart initiating the heartbeat. Therefore, the intrinsic

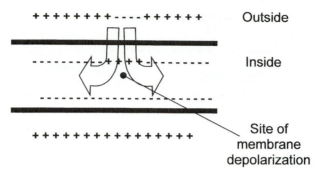

Figure 2–5
Depolarization spreads within a cell because positive charge flows to adjacent areas of negative charge.

beating rate of the heart is defined by the rate at which atrial cells rhythmically and spontaneously increase the conductance of Na and Ca ions.

An action potential does not occur simultaneously everywhere on a cell but is *propagated* from the initiating site of membrane depolarization over the remainder of the cell membrane (see Figure 2–5). At the initiating site of depolarization, the inside of the cell has become more positively charged (depolarized) because of the influx of Na ions, for example. Some of this positive charge diffuses toward adjacent areas of negative charge causing these areas to depolarize above threshold. An action potential is then generated in these adjacent membrane areas and the process is repeated in the next adjacent area until the action potential has spread over the whole cell membrane.

Cell-to-Cell Transmission of an Action Potential

- Gap junctions are direct intercellular connections.
- Chemicals released from nerve endings induce an action potential in an adjacent cell.
- Chemical agents act on ligand-gated channels.

The action potential is an important means of communication for the body, that is, electrical communication. The other major form of communication is through hormones. The major advantages of electrical communication over hormonal communication is that electrical communication is rapid and localized. Hormones are generally released into the blood and are carried throughout the body, therefore having a diffuse site of action.

There are several ways by which action potentials can be passed from one cell to another. Cells in some organs (eg, cardiac muscle, intestinal smooth

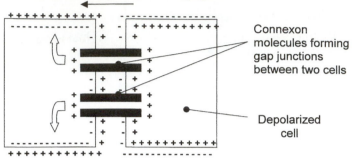

Figure 2–6
Depolarization spreads between cells by flowing through intercellular structures called gap junctions.

muscle, and uterine smooth muscle) are electrically connected through *gap junctions* (see Figure 2–6). Gap junctions are composed of a specialized protein called *connexon* that forms a pore through the cell membrane. Connexon molecules in one cell bind to connexon molecules in an adjacent cell so that the pores in each cell are aligned. The pairing of these pores prevents entry of material from outside the cell (the extracellular space) but allows materials from the inside of each cell (intracellular space) to exchange. Because ions can easily pass through gap junctions, an action potential in one cell will cause one to form in an adjacent cell because ions can move from the depolarized cell (the one having an action potential) to the one that is not. It is not clear which ion is involved in depolarizing an adjacent cell. As will be discussed in more detail later, the movement of the action potential from the sinoatrial node of the right atrium throughout the heart to produce each heart beat is possible because the heart cells are electrically connected through gap junctions.

An action potential can also be transmitted between cells by a chemical mediator. This is the primary mechanism by which nerve stimulation produces an action potential in an adjacent cell. The nerve action potential begins in the nerve cell body and travels down the axon of the nerve to the cell to be stimulated. At the end of the axon is a collection of vesicles that contain one or more chemicals called *neurotransmitters* (see Figure 2–7). When the action potential reaches the end of the axon, the depolarization causes Ca ions to enter the axon ending. This influx of calcium ions initiates a process through which the vesicles containing the neurotransmitter fuse with the axon membrane, open, and release the neurotransmitter to the exterior of the nerve cell. The neurotransmitter diffuses away from the nerve and binds to receptors on adjacent cells. When the neurotransmitter binds to a receptor, a signaling cascade is initiated that results in an increase in the conductance of Na and/or Ca channels. Activation of these ion channels initiates the movement of positive ions into the cell, the subsequent depolarization of the membrane potential above threshold, and an action potential. Because the

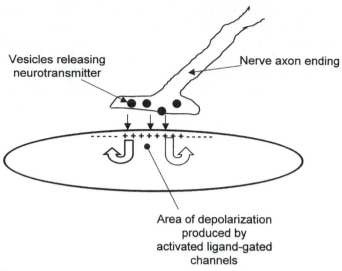

Figure 2–7
Nerves release chemical transmitters that diffuse to adjacent cells and depolarize the membrane by increasing the conductance to extracellular positive ions, usually Na and Ca.

binding of the neurotransmitter (ligand) to the receptor activates these ion channels, they are called *ligand-gated channels* to distinguish them from voltage-gated channels described previously. Nerve stimulation of cells can be very specific because specific nerves release specific neurotransmitters and these transmitters bind to specific receptors on stimulated cells. Examples of this specificity are presented in later chapters when the control of each organ system is discussed. A more in-depth understanding of ligand–receptor interaction can be obtained by reading *Basic Concepts in Pharmacology,* 2nd edition, by Janet L. Stringer.

PERIPHERAL NERVOUS SYSTEM

General Organization of the Nervous System

- Nervous system is divided into three systems: central, peripheral, enteric.
- Peripheral system is further subdivided into somatic and autonomic.
- Autonomic is further subdivided into sympathetic and parasympathetic.
- Enteric nervous system is contained within the gastrointestinal tract.

The nervous system is divided into several subsystems based primarily on anatomical criteria. The first division is into the central and peripheral systems. The *central nervous system* consists of the brain and spinal cord while the *peripheral nervous system* includes all nerves that enter and leave the central nervous system. The central nervous system receives information from receptors located throughout the body. These receptors sense one of five types of information: (1) mechanical (stretch, pressure); (2) thermal; (3) pain *(nociceptors);* (4) light (electromagnetic): and (5) chemical. Signals from specific receptors can converge with other nerves into discrete areas of the brain to form *feedback controller* or *integration centers* (see chapter 1). Because these areas receive signals about specific organ systems or elicit specific responses, these brain areas have been given names reflective of these characteristics, for example, cardiovascular, respiratory, auditory, visual, or vomiting centers. In subsequent chapters the role of these integration centers in controlling function of specific organ systems will be described.

The peripheral nervous system carries information into and out of the central nervous system. Peripheral nerves entering the central nervous system are coming from specific sensory receptors located throughout the body and are called *afferent nerves*. Peripheral nerves leaving the spinal cord are termed *efferent nerves* because they ultimately end on some cell to produce an effect. Based on anatomical and functional characteristics, the peripheral efferent nerves are divided into two types: somatic and autonomic. *Somatic nerves* innervate the skeletal muscles of the body; *autonomic nerves* innervate cardiac and smooth muscle as well as glands. The cell bodies of both the somatic and autonomic nervous systems are within the spinal cord, but the axon leaving the somatic nerve cell extends all the way to the skeletal muscle cell while axons of autonomic nerves connect to a second nerve cell whose axon innervates the final tissue. The autonomic nervous system is further subdivided into the *parasympathetic* and *sympathetic nervous systems*. The characteristics of the autonomic nervous system will be described in more detail in the next section since it plays an important role in the regulation of many organ systems of the body.

The *enteric nervous system* is unusual in that it is contained within the gastrointestinal tract. Many gastrointestinal functions are regulated solely by the enteric nervous system. The enteric nervous system can also be considered a part of the autonomic nervous system because it innervates smooth muscles and glands, as do nerves of the autonomic nervous system. The characteristics of the enteric nervous system are described in detail in chapter 6, Gastrointestinal Physiology.

Autonomic Nervous System

- Autonomic nerves synapse before reaching the final tissue.
- Parasympathetic and sympathetic nerves can be distinguished by the length of their pre- and postganglionic nerves and the neurotransmitters they release.

(continued)

> (*continued*)
> • Neurotransmitters released by the autonomic nervous system act on nicotinic, muscarinic, and adrenergic receptors.
> • The adrenal medulla is considered part of the autonomic nervous system.

A characteristic of the autonomic nervous system is that the axon of the autonomic nerve cell body in the spinal cord does not extend all the way to the tissue innervated (eg, heart, smooth muscle, gland) but ends on a second nerve (see Figure 2–8). The connection between the axon of one nerve cell and the cell body of a second nerve is called a *synapse*. A collection of synapses is called a *ganglion*. Nerve fibers entering a ganglion are called *preganglionic nerve fibers* while those leaving a ganglion are called *postganglionic nerve fibers*. In the autonomic nervous system, it is the postganglionic nerve fiber that innervates the heart, smooth muscle, or gland cells.

The length of the pre- and postganglionic nerve fibers anatomically defines the two divisions of the autonomic nervous system. The axon from the cell body of a sympathetic nerve leaves the spinal cord and extends a short distance before it synapses with a second nerve. These synapses are clustered into ganglia that are either close to the spinal cord *(paravertebral ganglia)* or a short distance from the cord *(prevertebral ganglia)*. In contrast, the axon from the cell body of a parasympathetic nerve extends all the way to the tissue innervated before forming a synapse. The ganglia of parasympathetic nerves are located in the organs innervated. Therefore, the length of the pre- and postsynaptic nerve fibers characterizes sympathetic and parasympathetic nerves. Sympathetic nerves have short preganglionic and long postganglionic nerve fibers while parasympathetic nerves have long preganglionic and short postganglionic nerve fibers.

The sympathetic and parasympathetic nervous systems can also be distinguished by the anatomical location where the preganglionic fibers leave the central nervous system. Sympathetic preganglionic nerve fibers leave the spinal cord at the level of the thorax and abdomen, that is, between the thoracic and lumbar (T1–L3) levels of the spinal cord. In contrast, parasympathetic preganglionic nerve fibers leave the central nervous system at the level of the midbrain and medulla as cranial nerves III, VII, IX, and X (vagus nerve) and at the bottom or sacral level (S2–S4) of the spinal cord. Approximately 75% of all preganglionic parasympathetic nerve fibers leave the central nervous system in the X cranial or vagus nerve.

The neurotransmitters released by the postganglionic nerve fibers of the two branches of the autonomic nervous system also distinguish these two systems (see Figure 2–8). *Acetylcholine (ACh)* is the neurotransmitter released by the preganglionic nerve fibers in both branches. In the parasympathetic nervous system,

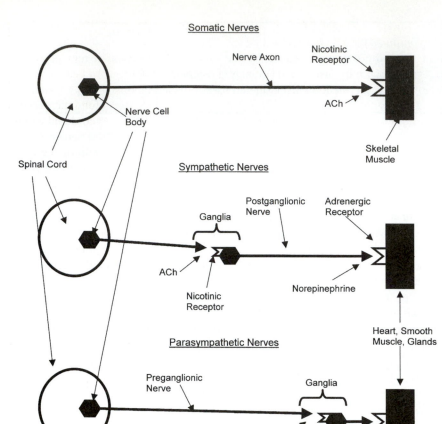

Figure 2–8
In this stylized drawing, the basic anatomical and pharmacological differences between
somatic, sympathetic, and parasympathetic nerves are illustrated.

acetylcholine is also released from the postganglionic nerve fiber; however, *nor-epinephrine (NE)* is released from the sympathetic postganglionic nerve fibers.

These neurotransmitters released by the autonomic nervous system act on
specific receptors (see Figure 2–8). Acetylcholine released by preganglionic
nerves acts on *nicotinic receptors* on the cell bodies of the postganglionic nerves.
Acetylcholine released from parasympathetic postganglionic nerve endings stimulates *muscarinic receptors* of the innervated tissue. Norepinephrine released
from sympathetic postganglionic nerve endings stimulates *adrenergic receptors*.
The muscarinic and adrenergic receptors can be further subdivided, but for our

purposes only the subdivisions of the adrenergic receptors will be considered here. Adrenergic receptors are subdivided into *alpha-adrenergic receptors* and *beta-adrenergic receptors*. The location of these receptors in the body and the tissue response to their stimulation will be described in subsequent chapters where their role in organ system function is described.

The *adrenal medulla* is considered a component of the autonomic nervous system. Some sympathetic preganglionic fibers leave the spinal cord and extend all the way to the adrenal medulla where they end on specialized neuronal cells that secrete *epinephrine* and *norepinephrine* (10:1, epinephrine:norepinephrine). Both epinephrine and norepinephrine are secreted into the blood stream, which enables them to circulate and stimulate adrenergic receptors throughout the body. Epinephrine stimulates both alpha and beta receptors. In a way, the adrenal medulla is analogous to the postganglionic sympathetic nerve fibers in that it releases hormones that stimulate adrenergic receptors. During activation of the sympathetic nervous system, the release of epinephrine from the adrenal medulla is an important component.

Somatic Nervous System

- Somatic nerves do not synapse before reaching the skeletal muscle cell.
- Somatic nerves release acetylcholine, which stimulates the nicotinic receptors on skeletal muscle cells.

As indicated above, axons of somatic nerves extend from the cell body in the spinal cord to the skeletal muscle cell without a synapse (see Figure 2–8). The nerve ending releases acetylcholine, which stimulates nicotinic receptors located on skeletal muscle cells causing them to contract.

MECHANISM OF MUSCLE CONTRACTION

Muscle Types

- Striated muscles derive their name from the striations seen under the microscope.
- Skeletal and cardiac muscle are striated muscles.
- Smooth muscles do not have striations when viewed under the microscope.
- Smooth muscles line hollow organs like blood vessels, the gastrointestinal tract, the uterus, and the bladder.

Muscles can be divided into two broad groups, striated and smooth, based on their appearance under light microscopy. *Striated muscles* include skeletal muscles responsible for body movement and cardiac muscle responsible for the pumping action of the heart. *Smooth muscle* is found in the walls of many structures including blood vessels, gastrointestinal tract, urinary bladder, and uterus.

Basis of Force Development

- Force is generated by thick-thin filament sliding.
- Myosin is in thick filaments; actin is in thin filaments.
- Myosin extensions from the thick filament to actin in the thin filament are called cross-bridges.
- Cross-bridges pull thin filaments past thick filaments.
- Myosin splits ATP and uses energy to move thin filaments.
- A specific intracellular Ca concentration is needed to stimulate actin-myosin interaction.

The basic process of muscle contraction is identical in both striated and smooth muscles. In both classes, contraction is initiated by an elevation in the intracellular Ca ion concentration produced by an action potential or chemical stimulus. The elevated intracellular Ca^{++} enables the two major contractile proteins *actin* and *myosin* to interact and generate force. It is the myosin molecule that is the "molecular motor" that converts chemical energy in the form of ATP to mechanical energy. When the intracellular Ca^{++} concentration returns to normal, the interaction between actin and myosin can no longer occur and the muscle relaxes.

Force is generated because myosin-containing *thick filaments* pull actin-containing *thin filaments* past them. The thin filaments ultimately attach to the cell membrane and enable the force generated by filament sliding to be transmitted to the surface of the cell. The sliding of thick and thin filaments occurs in the following way (see Figure 2–9). The portion of the myosin molecule containing an ATP splitting enzyme (ATPase) swings out from the thick filament and makes contact with actin in the thin filament. This extension from the thick filament is called a *cross-bridge*. When the cross-bridge contacts actin, ATP is split by the myosin ATPase located at the end of the cross-bridge. This provides only sufficient energy for the cross-bridge to slide the thin filament a discrete distance. After this movement, the cross-bridge separates from the thin filament, acquires another ATP, rebinds to another actin, and the cycle is repeated as long as there is sufficient Ca^{++} and ATP. In this way myosin "steps" from actin to actin along the thin filament, and the thin filament slides past the thick. Sliding is a smooth, continuous process because the cycling of the cross-bridges does not occur at the same moment; each cross-bridge cycles at a different moment. Because the actin

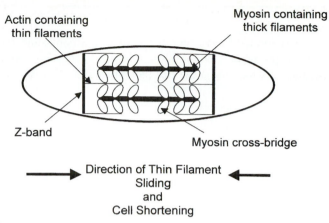

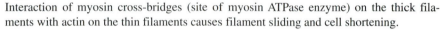

Figure 2–9
Interaction of myosin cross-bridges (site of myosin ATPase enzyme) on the thick filaments with actin on the thin filaments causes filament sliding and cell shortening.

thin filaments are attached to the membrane of the muscle cell, the cell shortens as thick and thin filaments slide past one another. Individual muscle cells are linked together by the connective material surrounding them so the shortening of each cell is transmitted throughout the tissue.

When we try to lift a weight, filament sliding produces force. If this sliding within the muscle can develop an amount of force equal to the size of the weight, the weight will be lifted and the muscle will shorten. This is called an *isotonic* contraction. The muscle is developing a constant amount of force (constant tension or isotonic) equal to the size of the weight it is lifting. However, if the weight is of such size that no amount of filament sliding will generate sufficient force to lift it, maximum force is produced but no shortening occurs. This is called an *isometric* contraction. The external length of the muscle does not change (constant length or isometric), and maximum force is developed.

Control of Intracellular Ca^{++} Concentration

- The intracellular Ca^{++} concentration is the determinant of contractile activity.
- Sarcoplasmic reticulum is an intracellular Ca^{++} store from which Ca^{++} can be released by chemical and electrical stimulation.
- Transverse tubules are membrane areas that carry electrical stimulation into the interior of the cell.

(continued)

(*continued*)
- Ca^{++} pump is located in the membrane of the sarcoplasmic reticulum (SR) and transports Ca^{++} into the SR.
- Ca^{++} channels are located on the cell membrane and allow Ca^{++} to enter the cell.
  - Voltage-gated Ca^{++} channels open in response to electrical stimulation.
  - Ligand-gated Ca^{++} channels open in response to chemical stimulation.

The intracellular Ca ion concentration is the essential determinant of contractile activity. In a noncontracting, resting muscle cell, the intracellular ionic Ca concentration is between 10^{-9} and 10^{-8} M. Stimulation of a muscle cell, either by an action potential or chemical stimulus, causes the Ca^{++} concentration to increase 100X. As the Ca^{++} concentration rises, more and more myosin molecules interact with actin, and the amount of shortening and force produced increases. When the action potential passes or the chemical stimulus is lost, the intracellular Ca^{++} concentration returns to resting levels, myosin can no longer interact with actin, thick and thin filaments return to their original position and the muscle lengthens.

Since the intracellular concentration of Ca^{++} plays such a critical role in controlling force development, muscle cells have a variety of mechanisms for its regulation. The sources of Ca^{++} are extracellular stores, intracellular stores, or both. Skeletal muscle uses primarily intracellular Ca^{++} stores, cardiac muscle uses a combination of both, and smooth muscle uses primarily extracellular stores. These differences are related to the size and speed with which muscle cells contract. Skeletal muscle cells are large and contract rapidly because of a rapid myosin ATPase. So diffusion of Ca^{++} from outside the cell, a relatively slow process, would not provide sufficient Ca^{++} rapidly enough to optimize the contractile potential of skeletal muscle. Therefore, skeletal muscle makes use of intracellular Ca^{++} stores contained within a vesicular structure called the *sarcoplasmic reticulum (SR)* (see Figure 2–10). The SR surrounds bundles of thick and thin filaments like a sleeve surrounds an arm. Because of the close physical proximity between the SR and the contractile filaments, Ca^{++} released from the SR is immediately available to initiate actin–myosin interaction. At intervals along the surface of a skeletal muscle cell, the cell membrane dips into the interior of the cell like a finger pushed into a balloon forming narrow, blind sacs called *transverse tubules* or *T-tubules.*

T-tubules pass very close to the SR to which they are electrically coupled. This coupling occurs through two receptors, one in the T-tubule, the *dihydropyridine receptor (DHP receptor),* and the other located in the SR, the *ryanodine receptor (RYR receptor).* The names of these receptors are derived from the names of the substances that bind to them. The RYR receptor looks like a mushroom

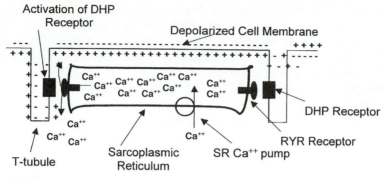

Figure 2–10
Muscle contraction is initiated by release of Ca^{++} from the sarcoplasmic reticulum. This release is initiated by a wave of membrane depolarization that travels down the T-tubule activating DHP receptors and opening the RYR receptors on the SR. Ca^{++} leaves the SR through the RYR receptors and activates the contractile proteins. After the cell membrane repolarizes, Ca^{++} is returned to the SR by an active transport system (Ca^{++} pump).

with the stem stuck into the SR and the cap protruding from the surface of the SR. Penetrating the receptor from cap to stem is a channel through which Ca^{++} can pass from the interior of the SR into the cytoplasm of the cell. Acetylcholine released from somatic nerves stimulates the nicotinic receptor on the skeletal muscle cell that initiates an action potential. The action potential travels along the muscle cell membrane and passes into the interior of the cell along the T-tubule activating DHP receptors. By an unknown mechanism, the activated DHP receptor opens the Ca^{++} channel in the RYR receptor allowing Ca^{++} to leave the SR and initiate actin–myosin interaction. Ca^{++} leaves the SR by passive diffusion because its concentration is greater in the SR than in the cell cytoplasm. The high SR Ca^{++} concentration is the result of a carrier protein located in the SR membrane that uses the energy from ATP (a Ca-ATPase) to transport Ca^{++} from the cell cytoplasm into the SR. When the RYR receptor is closed, the SR Ca-ATPase moves any released Ca^{++} from the cytoplasm back into the SR, reducing the amount of Ca^{++} available to initiate actin–myosin interaction and enabling the muscle to relax.

Cardiac muscle makes use of Ca^{++} coming into the cell during an action potential to induce the release of additional Ca^{++} from intracellular stores. The DHP receptor of cardiac muscle is a voltage-sensitive channel and when activated by the action potential, it opens and permits the entry of Ca ions. These Ca ions then activate RYR receptors on cardiac SR initiating the release of large quantities of Ca^{++} from the SR. After the action potential passes, the Ca-ATPase of cardiac SR moves the released Ca^{++} back into the SR lowering the cytoplasmic Ca^{++} concentration and permitting relaxation. Cardiac muscle cells also lower intracellular Ca^{++} concentration by a Na_o–Ca_i antiporter. Extracellular Na^+ moving into the cell down its concentration gradient drives the movement of intracellular Ca^{++} out of the cell. The release of SR Ca^{++} and its reuptake by the SR Ca ATPase and removal by the Na-Ca exchanger must occur within a fraction of a second so that the human heart can contract and relax 70 times a minute while at rest and even faster as heart rate increases.

Because of the small size of smooth muscle and its slow rate of contraction, diffusion of Ca^{++} from the extracellular space is generally adequate to supply sufficient Ca^{++} rapidly enough. However, some smooth muscle cells also contain a less developed SR that releases and takes up Ca^{++} following stimulation. This is especially true of smooth muscle found in arteries. Many biologically important substances have been shown to initiate smooth muscle contraction (eg, norepinephrine) by causing the release of Ca^{++} from smooth muscle SR or to produce relaxation by stimulating the uptake of Ca^{++} by the SR Ca-ATPase (eg, nitric oxide).

Ca^{++} Regulation of Actin–Myosin Interaction in Striated Muscle

- Basic mechanism involves removal of an inhibitor.
- Tropomyosin on thin filament prevents actin–myosin interaction.
- Ca^{++} binding to troponin removes tropomyosin inhibition.
- Actin–myosin interaction is permitted and force is generated.

Even though force development in both striated and smooth muscle is regulated through changes in intracellular Ca^{++}, the mechanism of this regulation is dramatically different. In striated muscle (skeletal and cardiac), Ca^{++} regulates force development by acting on proteins associated with the thin filaments while in smooth muscle, Ca^{++} interacts with proteins associated with the thick filaments.

In striated muscle, the thin filament contains two other proteins, *tropomyosin* and *troponin*, in addition to actin (see Figure 2–11). Under resting conditions (low Ca^{++}), tropomyosin physically prevents myosin from interacting with actin by covering the myosin-binding site on actin. This inhibition is removed when Ca^{++} binds to troponin. Troponin binds to actin and to tropomyosin. When Ca^{++} binds to troponin, this induces a conformational change in troponin that is transferred to tropomyosin causing tropomyosin to move away from the myosin binding sites on actin. With tropomyosin moved out of the way, myosin can bind to actin. Therefore in striated muscle, Ca^{++}, through the troponin–tropomyosin complex on the thin filament, removes an inhibition.

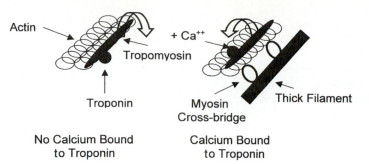

Figure 2–11

Ca^{++} activates skeletal muscle contractile proteins by binding to troponin, which causes a conformational change in tropomyosin. Because of the conformational change, sites on actin are exposed enabling myosin cross-bridges to bind and force to be generated.

Ca^{++} Regulation of Actin–Myosin Interaction in Smooth Muscle

- Basic mechanism involves activation of myosin.
- Ca^{++} activates myosin light-chain kinase.
- Activated myosin light-chain kinase adds a phosphate to the light chain of myosin and in the process activates myosin.
- Phosphorylated myosin interacts with actin-generating force.

Smooth muscle does not contain troponin so Ca^{++}, working through the thick filament, activates myosin rather than removes an inhibition. This occurs through an enzyme called *myosin light-chain kinase (MLCK)* (see Figure 2–12). Myosin light-chain kinase is an enzyme that takes a phosphate molecule from ATP and attaches it to a portion of the myosin molecule called the *light chain*. The light chain affects the shape of the myosin molecule and the activity of the myosin ATPase. When the light chain is phosphorylated, myosin becomes activated. Myosin attaches to actin in the thin filament and myosin ATPase metabolizes ATP. As long as the light chain is phosphorylated, actin–myosin interaction occurs, myosin ATPase splits ATP, cross-bridges cycle, and force is generated just as in striated muscle.

This is where Ca^{++} comes in because it is responsible for controlling the activity of myosin light-chain kinase and, therefore, the phosphorylation of the light chain. Calcium activates myosin light-chain kinase through its interaction with a protein called *calmodulin (CaM)*. Ca^{++} binds to calmodulin, the complex binds to myosin light-chain kinase, and the kinase becomes activated. The more

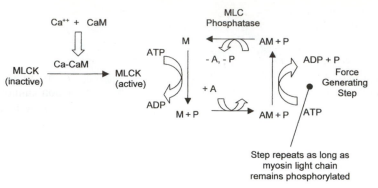

Figure 2–12
In contrast to striated muscle, activation of smooth muscle myosin requires phosphorylation of myosin light chain. Ca^{++} binding to calmodulin (CaM) activates myosin light chain
kinase (MLCK), the enzyme that catalyzes this phosphorylation (M + P). In the phosphorylated form, myosin can bind to actin and generate force.

Ca^{++}, the more Ca-calmodulin complex is formed, the more myosin light-chain
kinase is activated up to some maximum Ca^{++} level. If the Ca^{++} level is reduced,
the amount of Ca-calmodulin complex decreases and myosin light-chain kinase
activity falls. Finally, there is another enzyme, *myosin light-chain phosphatase
(MLCP)*, which is responsible for removing the phosphate from the light chain.
So the amount of light-chain phosphorylation at any time is determined by activities of myosin light-chain kinase and myosin phosphatase. The activity of both
the myosin light-chain phosphatase and kinase are regulated by various activa-
tors and inhibitors of smooth muscle contraction.

Two Fundamental Mechanical Relationships

- Length-tension relationship is dependent on muscle stretched-length.
- Most muscles are at their optimal stretched-length for forced develop-
  ment.
- Force development is determined by thick and thin filament overlap and
  Ca^{++} sensitivity.
- Force–velocity is an inverse relationship.
- Maximum shortening velocity is a measure of myosin ATPase activity.
- Force developed by myosin cross-bridge influences myosin ATPase
  activity.

Even though Ca^{++} is the essential regulator of contraction, the magnitude of force
development is also dependent upon the stretched-length of the muscle. This is

called the *active length-tension relationship* (see Figure 2–13). Changes in muscle stretched-length affect the magnitude of force development in three ways. One way involves the relative position of thick and thin filaments at the time Ca^{++} is released. There is an amount of overlap between thick and thin filaments that allows for optimal interaction between actin and myosin molecules. If the filaments are pulled too far apart or interdigitate too much, optimal interaction cannot occur. The extent of thick and thin filament overlap is determined by how relaxed or stretched a muscle cell is prior to stimulation. The second way stretched-length influences force involves changes in the effectiveness of Ca^{++} to activate actin-myosin interaction. As a muscle cell is stretched, it becomes thinner, causing the thick and thin filaments to move closer together. Because the filaments are closer, when Ca^{++} is released it is more effective in activating myosin, and the magnitude of force development increases. The final effect that stretch has is to change the amount of Ca^{++} released during muscle stimulation. Stretching muscle deforms the cell membrane and enhances the amount of Ca^{++} released with each stimulation. Because of this increase in Ca^{++} release, more force is developed.

Both striated and smooth muscles exhibit the active length–tension relationship and most muscles are at their optimal stretched-length for force development. An important exception is cardiac muscle. Cardiac muscle normally is at a length shorter than the optimal length. This is good because that means that if the heart fills more, its muscle cells will be at a longer stretched-length and it will contract more forcefully to eject the additional blood. The role the cardiac length-tension relationship plays in influencing cardiac output is discussed in detail in chapter 3, Cardiovascular System.

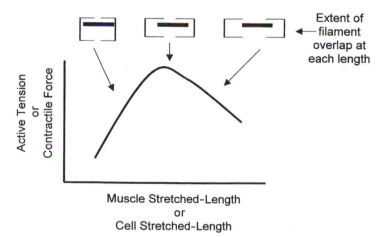

Figure 2–13
Different amounts of overlap between thick and thin filaments affect the amount of force a muscle can develop.

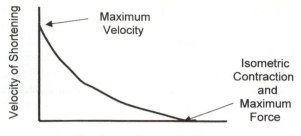

Figure 2–14
The velocity at which a muscle shortens decreases as the amount of force generated by the muscle increases. Light loads can be lifted faster than heavier loads.

There is an inverse relationship between how fast a muscle is able to shorten and how much force it can develop. This is called the *force–velocity relationship* (see Figure 2–14). Practical experience indicates that this relationship is correct because the heavier the weight you try to lift the slower you can do it. At the extreme, when you apply your maximum strength to lift a weight but cannot, the speed at which you lift the weight is zero.

The molecular basis of the force–velocity relationship can be understood by first examining the determinants of velocity and force. The velocity of muscle shortening is determined by the rate at which myosin cycles on and off actin. This cycle rate depends upon how rapidly myosin metabolizes ATP, which is equivalent to the myosin ATPase activity or the cross-bridge cycling rate. Myosin ATPase activity is genetically determined and varies between muscle types. In very broad terms, the myosin ATPase activity of muscles can be ranked as follows: skeletal > cardiac > smooth. On the other hand, the amount of force developed is related to the number of actin–myosin interactions occurring at any moment, which is equivalent to the number of cross-bridges formed at that moment. Therefore, the force–velocity relationship indicates that there is an inverse relationship between cross-bridge cycling rate (velocity) and the number of cross-bridges formed (force).

Since the myosin ATPase activity is genetically determined, the decreasing shortening velocity with increasing force must mean that the intrinsic velocity of the myosin ATPase must be altered as the muscle lifts increasing loads. This occurs because the myosin ATPase and the physical site at which myosin makes contact with actin are located close to one another on the end of the myosin molecule. As the weight the muscle is trying to lift increases, the amount of force each of these actin–myosin attachment sites must support also increases. This added force is transferred to the myosin ATPase site altering its conformation so that it metabolizes ATP slower. Because the cycling rate decreases due to the slower myosin ATPase activity, more cross-bridges will exist at any moment and the force developed will be greater.

CARDIOVASCULAR SYSTEM

·

GENERAL PRINCIPLES
Major Divisions of the Cardiovascular System

- Pulmonary circulation sends blood from right ventricle to left atrium.
- Systemic circulation sends blood from left ventricle to right atrium.
- The circulation systems are arranged in series.

The cardiovascular system is divided into the pulmonary and systemic circulations. These two circulations are arranged in *series* that is, blood flows first through one before it flows through the next. The *right ventricle* is the pump responsible for generating the pressure to move the blood through the pulmonary circulation. The *pulmonary circulation* carries blood through the lungs where it picks up oxygen and releases carbon dioxide. After passing through the lungs it returns to the *left atrium*. Blood from the left atrium flows into the *left ventricle*, which is the pump responsible for generating the pressure to move the blood through the systemic circulation. The *systemic circulation* carries this freshly oxygenated blood through the rest of the body. After passing through the body, the blood returns to the *right atrium* before being pumped once again by the right ventricle back through the lungs.

Organization of the Systemic Circulatory System

- Systemic circulation is organized into parallel circuits.
- Systemic circulation permits distribution of blood flow to specific organs.
- Blood flow to brain and heart is maintained over that to other organs during periods of reduced systemic arterial pressure.

The systemic arterial pressure is held constant to ensure adequate blood flow to the heart and brain. The systemic circulation is organized so that blood is delivered to all organs of the body simultaneously, that is, organized in *parallel circuits*. Parallel circuits enable the body to distribute flow where it is needed most and to maintain systemic arterial pressure. The public water system of your town is also organized in parallel circuits. Each house is attached to a central water line and the city maintains sufficient pressure so that water flows to every home. In a similar way, the organs of the body (eg, kidney, intestines, skeletal muscle) are each connected to the main blood vessel, the *aorta* (the blood vessel into which the left ventricle pumps). As long as the mean systemic arterial pressure (the pressure in the aorta) is maintained at the set point (approximately 100 mm Hg), each organ will receive adequate flow. However, there are situations, say during a draught, when the city limits water use and you can water your lawn or wash your car only on specific days. The same thing happens in the body. There are situations (eg, hemorrhage, heart failure) when the cardiovascular system cannot maintain the systemic arterial pressure at the set point. When this happens, blood flow is reduced. One way to correct this problem is to restrict flow to some organs just like the city restricts your water use. Flow is restricted in the body by increasing the resistance of vessels leading to specific organs. Blood flow to the heart and brain are essential for survival, so blood flow to other organs is preferentially reduced. By redirecting flow to critical organs the body also optimizes the use of the available blood volume. The available volume becomes more effectively used.

Vasculature

- Vasculature is divided into arterial, capillary, and venous components.
- Arterial walls consist of smooth muscle and endothelial cells.
- Arterioles, the smallest arterial subdivision, are the site of resistance control.
- Capillary walls consist only of endothelial cells.
- Capillaries are the site of fluid, nutrient, and waste exchange between blood and tissue.

(continued)

(*continued*)
• Vein walls consist of smooth muscle and endothelial cells.
• Veins contain two thirds of the blood volume so serve as a blood reservoir.

Blood leaves the ventricles through *arteries*, passes through the *capillaries,* and returns to the heart through *veins*. Arteries have thick walls composed of smooth muscle and endothelial cells and bands of elastic material composed of *elastin* and *collagen*. The thick walls enable them to resist the high pressure generated by the pumping action of the ventricles. Arteries branch many times with the final branch being the arterioles. The *arterioles* are the site of resistance control. Capillaries are differentiated from arterioles in that the walls of capillaries do not contain smooth muscle cells. Capillary walls consist only of a single layer of *endothelial* cells, which enables exchange of fluid, nutrients, and waste products with the surrounding tissue. Blood leaves capillaries through small veins called *venules*, which combine into ever-larger veins that carry the blood back to the heart. Veins contain fewer smooth muscle cells and elastin and collagen than do arteries of similar diameter. The venous system contains approximately two thirds of the total blood volume and serves as a blood reservoir. When this blood is needed, the smooth muscle cells in the walls of veins contract and reduce their diameter. This displaces blood into the arterial side of the circulation. Valves in the veins prevent blood from flowing away from the heart and break the column of blood into short segments reducing venous pressure.

Maintenance of Blood Pressure

• Generating pressure is the main function of the cardiovascular system.
• Systemic arterial pressure is a regulated variable.
• Baroreceptors, located in large arteries, are the sensors that monitor the systemic arterial pressure.
• The cardiovascular center, located in medullary region of the brain, is the integration center.
• The autonomic nervous system and the tissue it innervates is the effector system.

The main purpose of the cardiovascular system is to generate a pressure gradient so that blood flows throughout the vasculature delivering nutrients and removing metabolic waste products. Pressure is the regulated variable (see Homeostasis in chapter 1) of the cardiovascular system. Sensors *(baroreceptors)* monitor pressure and send information to the integrating center *(cardiovascular center)* located in the brain medulla. If pressure deviates from the set point, effector systems are activated to bring pressure back in line. The primary effector system is the autonomic nervous system and the tissues that it innervates, which include the vasculature, heart, kidney, and adrenal medulla.

The pressure that is monitored by the body is the pressure in large vessels of the systemic circulation. This is the *systemic arterial pressure*. Baroreceptors are located in the walls of large vessels (aorta and carotid arteries) close to the output of the left ventricle. The systemic arterial pressure is the same pressure recorded when you have your blood pressure taken. Systemic arterial pressure is usually reported as two values, the maximum pressure, *systolic pressure*, and the minimum pressure, *diastolic pressure*. Normal systolic pressure is 120 mm Hg and normal diastolic pressure is 80 mm Hg. Systolic pressure results from a new volume of blood being pumped into the systemic circulation with each contraction of the ventricle. Because the ventricle must refill before the next contraction, systemic arterial pressure declines to a minimum value, diastolic pressure, as blood flows throughout the circulation. Baroreceptors are sensitive to both the magnitude of systolic pressure as well as the difference between systolic and diastolic pressures, *pulse pressure*. Between any two heart beats, the time it takes to reach systolic pressure is about one third as long as the time it takes to reach diastolic pressure. Therefore, *mean arterial pressure (MAP)* is not the average of systolic and diastolic pressures but is described by this equation:

MAP = Diastolic pressure + One third pulse pressure

Determinants of Blood Flow

- Flow = Pressure gradient / Resistance.
- Pressure difference or gradient must exist for flow to occur.
- Resistance is determined by vessel radius, vessel length, and blood viscosity.
- Vessel radius is the most important regulator of resistance because resistance changes as the fourth power of the radius.

Knowing the relationship among flow, pressure, resistance, and volume is critical to understanding regulation of the cardiovascular system. The relationship among pressure, flow, and resistance is described by the following equation:

Flow = Pressure gradient / Resistance
or
$$F = (P_1 - P_2) / R \qquad \text{(equation 1)}$$

Flow occurs from a high pressure to a low pressure that is, down a *pressure gradient*, $P_1 - P_2$ in (equation 1). The greater the difference in pressure between two points, the greater will be the flow. In the body, blood flows from the ventricles to the atria. It is the pressure gradient between the ventricle and the atria that determines the magnitude of flow. For the pulmonary circulation this is the pressure difference between the right ventricle and the left atrium. For the systemic circulation this is the pressure difference between the left ventricle and the right atrium. Because the pressures in the atria are small, generally they are assumed to be zero and so only the pressures in the ventricles are considered. Finally, we are most often concerned with flow in the systemic circulation, so the pressure that determines flow in the systemic circulation is the mean arterial pressure. So we generally assume that flow is directly related to the magnitude of the mean arterial pressure. However, it must be remembered that this is just a simplification and that it is the pressure difference that determines flow.

For any given pressure gradient, flow is inversely related to the *resistance* to flow. Resistance to flow through blood vessels is determined by a variety of factors that include the length of the vessel, the radius of the vessel, and the viscosity of the blood. These factors are expressed in the following equation for resistance (R) developed by the 18th century French physician, Poiseuille:

$$R = (\eta \times l \times 8) / (\pi \times r^4)$$

In this equation, η is the viscosity of the blood, l is the vessel length, π is pi, and r is the radius of the vessel. An increase in vessel length or viscosity or a decrease in radius will raise resistance and reduce flow. Of these three, it is the radius of the vessel that is most critical for two reasons. One reason is that mathematically, resistance changes as the radius changes to the fourth power. This means that very small changes in radius will produce large changes in resistance. The second reason is that radius is the variable that the body easily changes to alter resistance. Because the vessel wall contains smooth muscle cells arranged helically, when these cells are made to contract or relax, the radius of the vessel will decrease or increase, respectively. Therefore, changes in vascular smooth muscle cell contractile activity will influence vascular resistance and, therefore, blood flow.

Blood Volume

• Blood volume is a regulated variable.
• Volume sensors are located in large venous vessels and heart.
• Blood volume is an important determinant of systemic arterial pressure.

Another factor influencing blood pressure and therefore flow is *volume*. The circulatory system is essentially a closed system containing a volume of blood equal to approximately 5 liters or 8% of the body weight (in kilograms). If this volume decreases, blood pressure will fall (assuming no other changes), and if volume increases, pressure will rise. Therefore, blood volume is an important determinant of blood pressure and blood flow. Blood volume is also a regulated variable. Sensors located in large veins entering the heart, the pulmonary artery, and the right atria of the heart monitor volume and, through homeostatic reflex systems, initiate responses to prevent changes in volume.

PUMPING ACTION OF THE HEART

Function of the Ventricles

> * Ventricles generate pressure gradient, which produces blood flow.
> * Cardiac output is the amount of blood pumped by a ventricle in a period of time.
> * Cardiac output of right and left ventricles must be equal since the pulmonary and systemic circulations are in series.

The right and left ventricles are responsible for generating a pressure gradient in the pulmonary and systemic circulations, respectively, so blood flow occurs. If they stopped pumping, there would be no pressure gradient and the pressure throughout the circulatory system would fall to about 7 mm Hg. This pressure, called the *mean circulatory pressure*, results from the elastic recoil of the blood vessel walls stretched by the volume of blood contained within them. So, the volume of blood pumped by each ventricle is critical to establish a pressure gradient and produce blood flow. The volume pumped by either ventricle per unit of time is called the *cardiac output (CO)* and averages about 5 L/min. Because the pulmonary and systemic circulations are in series, the CO of the right and left ventricles must be equal.

Since the CO is the output of the ventricles, it also represents the rate at which blood flows through the cardiovascular system and can be substituted for flow in equation 1 above. Also, as previously discussed, MAP is an approximation of the pressure gradient across the systemic arterial circulation, so (equation 1) can be rewritten and rearranged as follows:

$$CO = MAP/R \qquad \text{or} \qquad MAP = CO \times R$$

This equation describes the means by which the body regulates MAP, that is, by adjusting CO and R. In the next several sections, how the body controls CO will be discussed, and in later sections, the control of vascular resistance will be examined.

Cardiac Cycle

- Cardiac cycle is the events occurring during a single heartbeat.
- Cardiac cycle includes electrical and mechanical events.
- A single cycle requires less than 1 second to complete.

The *cardiac cycle* (Figure 3–1) is the sequence of events that occurs during one heartbeat and represents the coordination of electrical and mechanical events. It is divided into two phases, systole and diastole. In general, *systole* is the period during which the heart is contracting and ejecting blood, and *diastole* is the

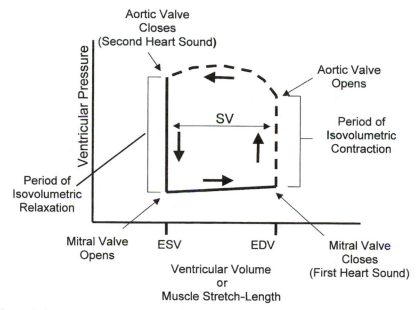

Figure 3–1
The sequence of events during a single contraction-relaxation cycle of the left ventricle can be depicted as a pressure volume curve as shown in this drawing. The pressure in the ventricle is plotted as a function of ventricular volume. As the left ventricle fills with blood, its volume increases from the volume at the end of systole (ESV) to the volume at the end of diastole (EDV). Ventricular contraction closes the mitral valve and causes pressure to rise rapidly (isovolumetric contraction) until it exceeds the pressure in the aorta. As soon as the aortic valve opens, blood is ejected from the ventricle causing the volume to decrease. The volume ejected with each beat is the stroke volume (SV), that is, the difference between EDV and ESV. During muscle relaxation, ventricular pressure falls (isovolumetric relaxation) until it is less than left atrial pressure, allowing the mitral valve to open and filling to begin again.

period when the heart is relaxing and filling with blood. At an average resting heart rate of 70 beats/min, 1 cardiac cycle is completed in less than a second (0.8 sec), and during strenuous exercise may last only a half a second or less as heart rate more than doubles. Because it is a cycle, one can start at any point so this discussion will begin at the moment when the ventricle begins to contract, that is, at the beginning of systole. For simplicity, events in the left ventricle will be described, but remember that similar events are occurring in the right ventricle simultaneously.

Systole

- Systole is the interval between the beginning of isovolumetric contraction and the end of ejection (indicated by a broken line in the cardiac cycle depicted in Figure 3–1).
- Systole lasts approximately one third of the cardiac cycle.
- Initially isovolumetric contraction occurs.
- Ejection begins when ventricular pressure exceeds aortic (or pulmonary artery) pressure and the aortic (or pulmonary artery) valve opens.
- Ejection continues until action potential has passed.
- End systolic volume is the ventricular volume at the end of ejection.

Systole begins at the moment when ventricular muscle is stimulated to contract by an action potential originating in the *sinoatrial node* of the right atrium. During the early period of systole, pressure rises within the left ventricle because of muscle contraction. The pressure is greater than in the left atrium so the valve between these two chambers (the *mitral valve*) closes, but it is not greater than the pressure in the aorta. Therefore, both the mitral and aortic valves are closed and the ventricle is contracting without changing volume, that is, it is contracting *isovolumetrically* or *isometrically*. Isovolumetric contraction continues until ventricular pressure exceeds aortic pressure. At this point the aortic valve opens and ventricular volume decreases as blood flows out into the aorta. As soon as blood leaves the ventricle, the period of isovolumetric contraction ends and the period of *ventricular ejection* begins. Ejection continues until the contraction of ventricular muscle cells ceases. This occurs when the action potential has spread throughout the ventricle. The interval between the beginning of isovolumetric contraction and the end of ejection is *systole*. The ventricular volume at the end of ejection is the *end systolic volume (ESV)*. The ventricle does not empty completely with each beat, therefore more blood can be ejected if the ventricle could be made to contract more forcefully. In subsequent sections we will see how this can happen.

Diastole

- Diastole is the interval from the beginning of ventricular relaxation to the beginning of ventricular contraction (indicated by a solid line in the cardiac cycle depicted in Figure 3–1).
- Diastole lasts approximately two thirds of the cardiac cycle.
- Initially it is a period of isovolumetric relaxation.
- Interval during which all ventricular filling occurs.
- End diastolic volume is the ventricular volume at the end of filling.

When contraction ends, ventricular muscle relaxes, which marks the beginning of *diastole*. As soon as the ventricular muscle begins to relax, pressure within the ventricle falls. This pressure is initially less than aortic pressure so the aortic valve closes, but the pressure in the ventricle is still greater than that in the left atrium, so the mitral valve remains closed. Since all valves are closed, relaxation occurs without a change in volume, that is, isovolumetrically. When ventricular pressure falls below atrial pressure, the mitral valve opens and ventricular filling begins. Filling continues until the ventricular muscle is stimulated to contract by an action potential. The ventricular volume at the end of filling is the *end diastolic volume (EDV)*.

FACTORS INFLUENCING THE PUMPING ACTION OF THE HEART

Cardiac Output

- $CO = SV \times HR = (EDV - ESV) \times HR = (mL/beat) \times (beats/min) = mL/min$.
- Stroke volume is the difference between end diastolic and end systolic volumes.
- Stroke volume is the volume per ventricular contraction (mL/beat).
- Heart rate measures contractions per unit of time (beats/min).

Cardiac output (CO) is determined by the volume of blood ejected by the ventricle with each beat (*stroke volume, SV*) and the number of times the ventricle contracts per unit of time (*heart rate, HR*). The stroke volume is the difference between the volume of blood in the ventricle just before it contracts (*end diastolic volume, EDV*) and the volume of blood at the end of contraction (*end systolic volume, ESV*). An increase (decrease) in either SV or HR will raise (decrease) CO.

Heart Rate

- Heart rate is initiated by action potentials from the SA node of the right atrium.
- SA node cells spontaneously depolarize (pacemaker potential) due to opening of Ca^{++} and Na^+ channels.
- Norepinephrine from sympathetic nerves increases heart rate by increasing the slope of the pacemaker potential.
- Acetylcholine from parasympathetic nerves decreases heart rate by decreasing the slope of the pacemaker potential.
- Epinephrine from the adrenal medulla increases heart rate by increasing the slope of the pacemaker potential.

The heart rate is determined by the spontaneous rate of membrane depolarization of the cells of the *sinoatrial (SA)* node located in the right atrium. Ion channels in the membranes of these specialized atrial cells allow Ca and Na to enter causing the cells to slowly depolarize. This slow depolarization is called the *pacemaker potential* (see Figure 3–2). When the membrane potential has decreased to the threshold potential, calcium channels open and an action potential is initiated as described in chapter 2. The action potential spreads rapidly by way of gap junc-

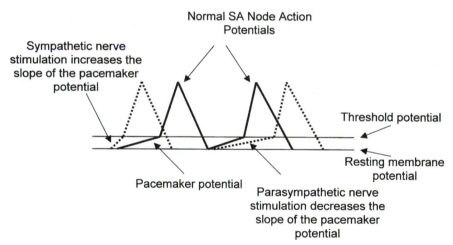

Figure 3–2
Spontaneous membrane depolarization of sinoatrial cells is altered by norepinephrine and acetylcholine released from sympathetic and parasympathetic nerve endings, respectively. By changing the rate of depolarization, sympathetic and parasympathetic nerve stimulation alter heart rate.

tions to all cells of the heart and initiates ventricular contraction (see Electrical Activity of the Heart, following, for more details).

The slope of the pacemaker potential determines the heart rate. The steeper the slope of the pacemaker potential, the faster the membrane potential decreases to threshold and the sooner an action potential occurs. Action potentials occur less frequently if the slope is more gradual. Postganglionic nerves of the two branches of the *autonomic nervous system, sympathetic* and *parasympathetic* (see chapter 2), innervate the SA node and influence the slope of the pacemaker potential. Sympathetic nerves release the neurotransmitter *norepinephrine (NE)* that stimulates *beta-1 adrenergic receptors* and increases the slope by opening more Ca^{++} and Na^+ channels. Therefore, sympathetic nerve stimulation increases heart rate and consequently increases CO. Postganglionic parasympathetic nerves release *acetylcholine (ACh),* which stimulates *muscarinic receptors* and reduces the number of open Ca^{++} channels as well as increases the opening of K channels. The net result is to reduce the slope of the pacemaker potential, slow heart rate, and reduce CO. Finally, the adrenal medulla releases *epinephrine* when stimulated by sympathetic nerves and epinephrine has the same effect on heart rate as norepinephrine.

In the absence of autonomic nervous system activity, the heart rate set by the rate at which the SA node generated action potentials would be about 80 beat/min. Since the normal heart rate at rest is approximately 70 beat/min the parasympathetic nervous system must be inhibiting the SA node to decrease the heart rate.

Stroke Volume

Four factors determine the magnitude of SV:
• End diastolic volume
• Ventricular contractility
• Ventricular afterload
• Heart rate

Four factors determine the magnitude of stroke volume. One factor that influences the pumping ability is end diastolic volume (EDV, see Figure 3–3). EDV sets the stretch-length of the ventricular muscle cells just before they contract at the beginning of systole. As described in chapter 2, changing muscle stretch-length through a variety of mechanisms influences the ability of myosin to generate force. At normal EDV, ventricular muscle is at a stretch-length that is shorter than the optimal for actin–myosin interaction and force development. Therefore, an increase in EDV will increase the stretch-length and enhance force

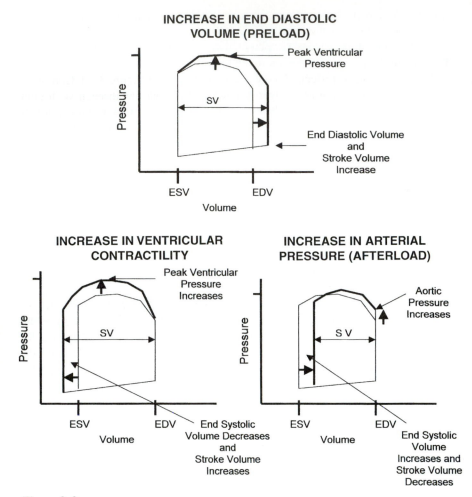

Figure 3–3
The impact of changes in preload, contractility, and afterload on stroke volume can be seen in these three left ventricular pressure-volume loops.

development, while a decrease in EDV will do the opposite. This property of ventricular muscle is called Starling's law of the heart and is very important for normal ventricular function. The right and left ventricles are connected in series, so whatever volume one ventricle pumps, has to be matched by the other. Balancing the output of the two ventricles occurs automatically because of the effect of EDV on ventricular force development. If the right ventricle pumps a larger volume into the left, the EDV of the left ventricle increases along with its ability to pump the larger volume so its output increases to match that of the right. Had the ventricles been at their optimal stretch-length, as are most muscles, an increase in EDV would result in a fall of force development and a reduction in pumping ability.

A second factor influencing SV is *contractility* (see Figure 3–3). Contractility is determined by the amount of calcium ions released with each ventricular action potential. If more (less) calcium is released, more (less) myosin is activated and more (less) force is generated at any stretch-length (EDV). Norepinephrine released from sympathetic nerves and epinephrine released from the adrenal medulla stimulate *beta-1 receptors* on ventricular muscle cells to increase the amount of calcium released with each action potential. This increases ventricular contractility and SV. The parasympathetic nervous system does not have a significant direct effect on ventricular contractility, but it does decrease atrial contractility by reducing the amount of Ca released with each action potential through the action of acetylcholine on muscarinic receptors.

The third factor influencing SV is *afterload* (see Figure 3–3). Afterload is the "load" or force against which the ventricle must pump. One form of afterload is the pressure in the pulmonary artery or aorta. For blood to leave the ventricles, the ventricles have to develop sufficient pressure to open the valves of the outflow vessels (aortic and pulmonic valves). These valves are kept closed by the pressure in the pulmonary artery or aorta. So, the ventricles must overcome the systemic arterial pressure or pulmonary artery pressure before ejection will begin. Therefore, these arterial pressures represent ventricular afterloads. Another form of afterload results from the tension in the ventricular wall. As in any hollow structure, as volume increases, tension (or force) in the wall increases. This tension acts to pull the wall apart. Think of an inflating balloon. As the ventricle fills with blood, the tension in the wall increases. When ventricular muscle cells contract, the force these cells develop acts against the wall tension produced by a particular EDV. This wall tension, therefore, is also an afterload. During the isovolumetric contraction phase of the cardiac cycle (see Figure 3–1), ventricular muscle generates force to overcome the afterload. The length of the systolic phase of the cardiac cycle is fixed by the duration of the action potential, so the greater the afterload, the longer the isovolumetric contraction phase has to be for the ventricle to develop the needed force. In addition, as the amount of force the ventricle needs to develop increases, the rate at which it develops this force decreases (remember the force–velocity relationship described in chapter 2). This also prolongs the isovolumetric phase. Therefore, as afterload (arterial pressure or EDV) rises, SV decreases.

The fourth determinant of SV is heart rate. Heart rate influences SV when the rate is very high (> 150 beat/min). Ventricular filling occurs during diastole (see Figure 3–1). At very high HR, this time is shortened and so there is less time for filling. This results in a decrease in EDV and the contractile ability of the ventricle.

ELECTRICAL ACTIVITY OF THE HEART

Action Potential Conduction

Action potential conduction proceeds along the following path: SA node–Atrial muscle–AV node–Bundle of His–Purkinje system–Ventricular muscle.

The SA node cells in the right atrium spontaneously generate action potentials as described in Heart Rate above. The action potential is conducted rapidly from these cells throughout the atrium and converges at the AV node, another group of specialized atrial cells located near the ventricles. Conduction through the atrium takes about 0.1 sec. AV node conduction is slow and requires another 0.1 sec to be completed. The slow conduction is because the upstroke of the action potential is due to an increase in Ca ion conductance, which is slow, compared to the rapid increase in Na ion conductance that occurs in the atrial cells. This produces a delay between the depolarization of the atria and the ventricles, which can be reduced or increased by sympathetic or parasympathetic nerve stimulation, respectively. Conduction then proceeds rapidly (0.1 sec) throughout the ventricle via the bundle of His and Purkinje system. The action potential is carried by the Purkinje system down the septum dividing right and left ventricles. It then moves up the walls proceeding from the inner to the outer surface of the ventricles. Because of this path, contraction begins at the bottom of the ventricles and progresses upward, forcing blood out the aorta or pulmonary artery located at the top of the ventricles.

Electrocardiogram

- Electrocardiogram is an external recording of the electrical activity of the heart.
- Shape of ECG trace depends on location of electrodes relative to conduction path through the heart.
- Magnitude of deflections is related to mass and orientation of the heart.

Electrocardiogram (ECG) is the external recording of the electrical activity of the heart. In the absence of an action potential, the outside of cells is positively charged relative to the inside (see chapter 2), therefore, the outside of the heart is positively charged. As the action potential passes over the heart, the outside of the cells and the outside of the heart become negatively charged. This cyclical change in external charge from positive to negative to positive again with the passing action potential is reflected in the ECG. Electrodes placed on the skin can detect these changes in charge on the heart because the body fluids conduct the changes to the skin.

The shape of the ECG trace depends upon the location of the skin electrodes relative to the conduction path of the cardiac action potential. Because the orientation of the heart and the conduction path of the action potential are fixed, electrodes placed at different locations will generate different ECG patterns. Twelve different electrode locations have been developed to assess electrical activity of the heart. However, if the orientation of the heart or the conduction path is changed from normal because of disease, the pattern of the ECG measured at one or more of these 12 electrode positions will be altered. Combining information from all leads can provide information about heart size, orientation within the chest, and the path of electrical conduction.

The magnitude of deflections in an ECG trace is related to the mass of the heart tissue undergoing a change in electrical charge. The electrical activity of the left ventricle, being the most massive portion of the heart, dominates the deflections in an ECG.

Components of a Typical ECG Trace

- Three major components of an ECG are P wave, QRS complex, T wave.
  —P wave: atrial depolarization
  —QRS complex: depolarization of ventricles
  —T wave: repolarization of ventricles
- PR interval is the interval from the beginning of atrial activation to the beginning of ventricular activation.
- QT interval is the time required for ventricular depolarization and repolarization.

A stylized ECG trace that might be recorded from the bipolar limb lead II (see next section for details) is illustrated in Figure 3–4. The first deflection represents atrial depolarization and is called the *P wave*. It is small in magnitude because the mass of the atria is small and it is short lived because all the atrial cells rapidly become depolarized. Once all atrial cells are depolarized, there is no charge difference across the atrial surface, so the ECG trace is flat. This is called the *isoelectric line*. The next deflection is the *QRS complex*. It is caused by depolarization of the ventricles and is large in magnitude because of their large mass. Again, when all ventricular cells have depolarized, there is no charge difference across the ventricular surface and the trace returns to the isoelectric line. The final deflection is the *T wave*, which reflects repolarization of the ventricles. Notice that there is no deflection reflecting repolarization of the atria. This is because atrial repolarization occurs at the time of ventricular depolarization and so is obscured by the large QRS complex.

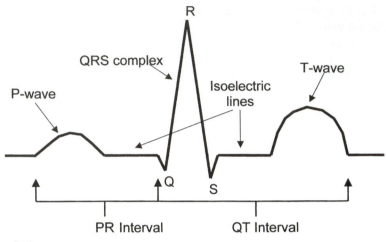

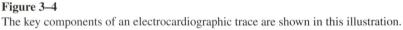

Figure 3–4
The key components of an electrocardiographic trace are shown in this illustration.

In addition to deflection patterns, two intervals provide useful information about heart function. The first interval is the *PR interval*. This is the time interval between the beginning of atrial depolarization and the beginning of ventricular depolarization. It is between 0.12 and 0.2 sec in duration. Most of the interval is the time required for action potential conduction through the AV node so changes in the length of this interval reflect change in AV-node conduction rate. The second interval is the *QT interval*. This is the time interval required to completely depolarize and repolarize the ventricles. It lasts about 0.4 sec.

Coordination of ECG and Cardiac Cycle

- P wave signals atrial contraction and the last of ventricular filling.
- QRS complex signals the end of diastole and the beginning of systole.
- T wave is the beginning of ventricular relaxation.
- QT interval represents the duration of systole.
- The first two heart sounds correspond to the closing of the mitral and aortic valves, which delineate the duration of systole.

Because the ECG reflects the electrical activity of the heart and, therefore, the contractile activity of the heart, the ECG is correlated with the cardiac cycle (see Figure 3–5). The P wave and atrial contraction signal the completion of ventricular filling as the last volume of blood is placed in the ventricle. From the PR interval we know that this final period of ventricular filling takes about 0.2 sec.

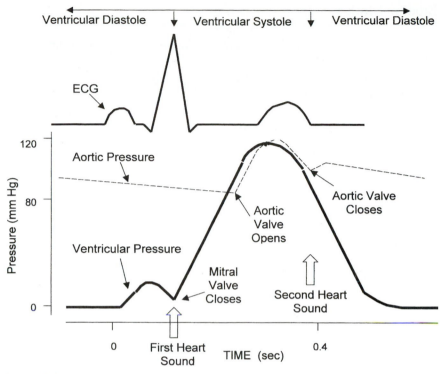

Figure 3–5
The electrical and pressure changes occurring within the cardiovascular system during a single contraction of the left ventricle are correlated in this drawing.

The QRS complex signals the contraction of the ventricles. This marks the end of diastole, the beginning of systole, and isovolumetric contraction. During the QRS complex and the subsequent period of complete ventricular depolarization (isoelectric line), the ventricles develop sufficient pressure to eject blood. The T wave, signaling ventricular repolarization, marks the beginning of ventricular relaxation. The force generated by the ventricles decreases and ejection is reduced. By the end of the T wave the ventricles are completely repolarized, systole ends, and isovolumetric relaxation begins. The QT interval, therefore, reflects the length of systole.

The "lub" (S_1) and "dup" (S_2) sounds heard with a stethoscope placed over the heart reflect the closing of the atrial-ventricular valves (mitral, tricuspid) and the semilunar (aortic and pulmonary) valves, respectively. The sounds are due to vibrations produced by the sudden closing of these valves. The closing of these two valves mark the beginning and end of systole and so the interval between them is a measure of the duration of systole.

Bipolar Limb Leads

- Bipolar limb leads measure electrical changes between two different limbs.
- The leads are: lead I: right arm (negative), left arm (positive); lead II: right arm (negative), left leg (positive); lead III: left arm (negative) , left leg (positive).
- Upward deflection of ECG trace indicates movement of electrical activity toward the positive electrode.
- Magnitude of deflections on ECG trace are not identical for all three leads because each has a different "view" of electrical conduction through the heart.
- Bipolar limb leads can be used to measure the orientation of the heart in the chest using Einthoven's triangle.

Electrodes used to generate ECG traces are divided into two general classes, *bipolar* and *unipolar limb leads* (see Figure 3–6). These in turn are further subdivided into three bipolar leads and nine unipolar leads.

The three bipolar limb leads measure the difference in electrical charge between two limbs: lead I—between the two arms; lead II—between the right arm and left leg; lead III—between the left arm and left leg. The location of the three limb leads defines the points of an equilateral triangle projected on the surface of the body called *Einthoven's triangle*, illustrated in Figure 3–6. By convention, leads are connected so that an upward deflection in the ECG trace occurs when the left arm or leg is positive relative to the right arm. As illustrated in Figure 3–6, the heart is oriented diagonally in the chest with the ventricles down and to the left. This means that the propagation of the cardiac action potential begins in the right atrium and moves downward and to the left as shown by the arrow.

To understand the ECG trace of any limb lead, it is important to remember that the leads sense changing electrical charge on the surface of the heart. Initially the outside of all heart cells is positive so the entire surface of the heart is positive and no leads sense a difference in charge. However, when an action potential begins in the SA node, the cells in this area become negative on the outside. This establishes a charge difference between atrial cells surrounding the SA node and the rest of the atrium (still outside positive) that sweeps across the atrium. The limb leads detect this moving charge difference. The right arm electrode is negative because it "sees" primarily the depolarized atrial cells near the SA node, while the left arm and left leg "see" primarily the remainder of the atrium, which is positive. This produces an upward deflection, by convention, in the ECG trace and represents the P wave. When the atria are completely depolarized (all cells outside negative), there is no charge difference across the surface, no moving wave of electrical charge, and so an isoelectric line is recorded (see PR interval in Figure 3–4). Even though no moving electrical charge is detected,

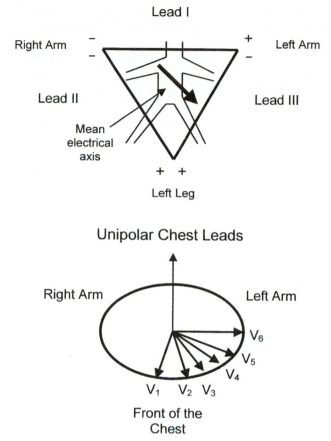

Figure 3–6
The bipolar limb leads (lead I, lead II, and lead III) detect electrical changes in the heart that can be used to calculate the mean electrical axis (arrow). Unipolar chest leads (V_1 to V_6) provide information about electrical conduction through specific regions of the heart.

the action potential is moving through the AV node and into the Purkinje fibers. This is not detected because the mass of tissue involved is too small to be sensed by the electrodes. The action potential next sweeps over the ventricles. Because of their large mass, there is a large charge difference between those portions of the ventricles that have been depolarized by the action potential and those that have not. This large charge difference accounts for the large magnitude of the QRS complex. Depolarization occurs from the inner ventricular surface *(endocardium)* to outer surface *(epicardium)* and moves from the bottom to the top of the ventricles. When the ventricles are completely depolarized, there is no difference in charge over the surface of the ventricles, no moving wave of depolarization, and a second isoelectric line is recorded. Repolarization of the ventri-

cles occurs in the opposite direction from depolarization beginning at the epicardium. Because of this reversal of direction, the T wave is recorded as a positive rather than a negative deflection.

The size of the P wave and QRS complex recorded in the three bipolar
limb leads is not the same. The reason for this is the relative positions of the
limb leads and the direction of action potential propagation over the heart.
The more the direction of electrical propagation points toward a positive limb
lead, the larger will be the ECG deflection. As illustrated in Figure 3–6, the
direction of propagation, as depicted by the arrow, points more directly at the
positive electrodes of leads I (left arm) and II (left leg) than at lead III. For
lead III the arrow points between the left arm and left leg. This means leads I
and II will "see" a greater charge difference between their two electrodes than
will lead III.

The differences in size of the QRS complex between the three bipolar limb
leads can be used to determine the orientation of the heart within the chest. If the
heart is positioned in the chest so that the ventricles point straight down, the
arrow describing the direction of electrical propagation will point at the positive
leg electrode. This will make the QRS deflections in leads II and III very large
and the QRS in lead I small. In this situation, the direction of propagation is essentially perpendicular to lead I. Therefore, this lead does not register much of a
difference between the positive and negative electrodes. Alternatively, if the heart
was oriented so that the ventricles point toward the left arm, the QRS deflection
will be large in lead I and small in leads II and III. In fact, the QRS in lead III
may be inverted since the direction of propagation is away from the positive electrode in this lead. One can imagine how the magnitude of the QRS complex in
the three limb leads would change if the heart assumed positions between these
extremes. By measuring the height of the QRS complex in the three bipolar
leads, you can calculate the orientation of the heart within the chest. How to do
this calculation is beyond the scope of this book.

Unipolar Limb Leads

- Unipolar limb leads measure charge differences between a positive exploring electrode and an indifferent negative electrode.
- Unipolar limb leads include six chest leads (precardial) designated V_1 to
  V_6 and three augmented limb leads designated aVR, aVL, and aVF.
- Chest and augmented leads are useful in diagnosing changes in ventricular mass.

Unipolar limb leads consist of a positive exploring electrode placed at specific
anatomical locations on the body and a negative, indifferent electrode. As with

the bipolar leads, unipolar leads measure the changing charge difference between the exploring electrode and the indifferent electrode.

One set of unipolar leads is the *six chest* or *precardial leads* (see Figure 3–6). These leads are placed on the chest starting just right of the sternum and moving down and to the left so that the sixth exploring electrode is placed on the chest below the armpit. These are designated V_1 to V_6. The QRS complex in each lead is different both in direction and magnitude because each exploring electrode has a different "view" of electrical conduction through the heart. The V_1 exploring electrode "views" the top right of the heart and normally electrical conduction is away from this exploring electrode so the QRS is negative (inverted). The QRS complex for exploring electrodes V_2 through V_6 becomes more positive as the position of the exploring electrode on the chest is more in line with the path of electrical conduction. Since the normal conduction path is down and to the left (see arrow in Figure 3–6), V_5 and V_6 have positive QRS complexes.

Chest leads are useful in detecting changes in ventricular mass because their anatomical position makes them dominated by specific ventricular chambers. Since ventricular mass influences the magnitude of the QRS complex, increased mass of ventricular tissue *(ventricular hypertrophy)* will be reflected in the size of the QRS complex. Lead V_1 is positioned over the right ventricle and is influenced by the electrical activity of this chamber. Leads V_5 and V_6 are at the bottom of the left ventricle and are influenced by this chamber. Therefore, if the magnitude of the QRS complex in V_1 increases this would be indicative of right ventricular hypertrophy, while an increase in V_5 and V_6 would indicate left ventricular hypertrophy.

There are also three *augmented limb leads.* Augmented limb leads consist of one of the limb leads (eg, right arm) compared to the two other leads (eg, left arm and left leg) combined into a single negative lead. By combining two limb leads into one, the charge difference between it and the exploring electrode is augmented, hence their name. The three exploring electrodes are designated aVL, aVR, and aVF indicating the position of the exploring electrode as the left arm (aVL), right arm (aVR), or left leg (aVF).

Augmented limb leads are also useful in assessing changes in ventricular mass. The right ventricle influences lead aVR, located on the right side of the body. Therefore, an increase in the magnitude of its QRS complex would be indicative of right ventricular hypertrophy. The QRS complex in leads aVL and aVF would be expected to increase with left ventricular hypertrophy since primarily the left ventricle influences them.

ROLE OF ARTERIAL RESISTANCE IN MAINTAINING BLOOD PRESSURE

In the beginning of this chapter it was stated that the purpose of the cardiovascular system was to generate a pressure gradient so that blood would flow throughout the body to deliver nutrients and remove waste products. The role of the heart in generating a pressure gradient has been described. In this section, the role of the vasculature will be described. The arterial system influences the pressure gradient by altering resistance while the venous system influences pressure by altering blood volume.

Impact of Arterial Resistance on Pressure and Flow

> • Arteriolar diameter is the major site of resistance control.
> • An increase in resistance decreases flow.
> • An increase in resistance increases the pressure gradient.

The arterioles form the site of major resistance control. Since resistance is related to the fourth power of the radius (see Determinants of Blood Flow above), a small change in arteriolar radius will have a dramatic effect on resistance.

As stated earlier, the relationship among flow, pressure, and resistance is described by the this equation:

$$Flow = Pressure\ gradient\ /\ Resistance$$

This equation indicates that an increase in resistance will decrease flow. This means that a decrease in arteriolar radius (an increase in resistance) will reduce flow. Also, if resistance increases, the pressure gradient must increase to produce the same level of flow.

Impact of Arterial Resistance on Cardiovascular System

> • Resistance changes to maintain a constant systemic arterial pressure.
> • Because of the parallel organization of the cardiovascular system, resistance changes result in redistribution of blood flow.

From a survival standpoint, the purpose of the cardiovascular system is to maintain adequate blood flow to the brain and heart. If systemic arterial pressure is inadequate to do this, homeostatic reflexes are initiated to elevate the pressure gradient so there is adequate blood flow. Because the circulatory system is organized into parallel circuits, the body can redirect blood flow to the heart and brain by restricting flow to other organs (eg, skin, kidneys, intestines). This is accomplished by increasing the resistance of arterioles supplying these organs. Because of the increased resistance, blood pressure within the organs falls while that in the rest of the circulation rises. So, an increase in arteriolar resistance selectively decreases blood flow to and pressure in specific organs, but results in the normalization of systemic arterial blood pressure thereby ensuring adequate blood flow to the brain and heart. This can be seen in the equation we examined before:

$$MAP = CO \times R$$

By increasing arteriolar resistance, MAP rises and the brain and heart are adequately perfused. Changes in arteriolar resistance can compensate for inadequate CO resulting from either an inability of the heart to pump or an inadequate blood supply.

Local Control of Arterial Resistance

Surrounding Tissue Alters Environment

> - Blood flow is matched to the metabolic needs of the tissue.
> - Mismatch between blood flow and metabolism leads to an altered chemical environment:
>   —Active hyperemia is an increase in blood flow to match an increase in metabolic activity.
>   —Reactive hyperemia is an increase in blood flow in response to a period of reduced flow.

A city water system is a useful analogy to understand local control of arteriolar resistance. The purpose of a city water system (in addition to providing adequate supplies of clean water) is to ensure an adequate water pressure so that when you open a faucet, water will flow out. If a house is equivalent to an organ of the body, then opening a faucet is the same as reducing the resistance of arterioles supplying an organ. This is local control of flow. You do not telephone the water department and ask them to open a faucet. You control that yourself. Also, one faucet being opened has minimal impact on the water pressure throughout the city. In the same way, changes in flow to an organ can usually occur without changing systemic arterial pressure.

In the circulatory system, local control of blood flow is mediated through changes in the concentration of local chemicals. The concentration of these substances is changed by changes in the metabolic activity of the tissue or by physically restricting flow to an organ.

The magnitude of blood flow is matched to the metabolic needs of the tissue by local chemical factors. If the metabolic activity of an organ increases, blood flow increases. This is called *active hyperemia*. When metabolic activity increases, there is a change in the local concentration of various chemicals that influences the resistance of arterioles. Substances such as oxygen decrease while carbon dioxide, hydrogen ions, and adenosine increase. These changes relax the smooth muscle cells in the arterioles, decrease resistance, and increase blood flow. The increase in flow provides more oxygen and washes away the excess carbon dioxide, hydrogen ions, and adenosine. A new balance is established between the concentration of these local chemicals and the blood flow. In a similar way, a fall in organ metabolic activity produces the opposite changes in concentration of these local chemicals. This will result in an increase in resistance and a fall in blood flow.

Active hyperemia may occur in a circumscribed set of tissues as when you wiggle one finger. This redirection of blood flow to your finger will not impact the flow in the rest of your body. However, if active hyperemia is extensive, as occurs in the skeletal muscles of a marathon runner, then flow to other organs of the body may be compromised.

If a physical restriction in blood flow produces a mismatch between flow and metabolic need, *reactive hyperemia* occurs. When the blood vessels into an organ are blocked, oxygen delivery is reduced and metabolic waste products (carbon dioxide, hydrogen ions, and adenosine) accumulate. These changes produce relaxation of arteriolar smooth muscle and a decrease in resistance. However, flow is prevented from increasing because vessels upstream from the arterioles are blocked. As soon as this blockage is released, there will be an immediate elevation in flow because the arterioles have dilated. The increase in flow is a reaction to the blockade. As the concentration of these local chemicals is returned to their normal levels, resistance will increase and flow will return to normal levels.

You have probably experienced reactive hyperemia. If you sit with your legs crossed for an extended time, large vessels in the dangling leg are physically blocked because of the weight of the leg. During this blockade, local chemicals decrease the resistance of arterioles in your leg muscles. When you uncross your legs, blood flow increases dramatically because of the low vascular resistance. If the blockade was of a long duration, a tingling sensation is also perceived when blood flow is restored, which is the feeling that your leg has "fallen asleep."

Endothelial Derived Factors Influence Vascular Resistance

> • Endothelial cells lining all blood vessels release factors that change vascular resistance.
> • Endothelial cells release nitric oxide in response to changes in blood flow velocity.

Endothelial cells that line all blood vessels play an important role in regulating local vascular resistance. Endothelial cells release a variety of substances that influence vascular resistance when stimulated by chemical and physical factors. A detailed description of the control of all endothelial-derived substances is beyond the scope of this book, so this discussion will focus on only one, the gas *nitric oxide (NO)*. Endothelial cells contain an enzyme called *nitric oxide synthase (NOS)* that catalyzes the formation of NO from the amino acid arginine. Nitric oxide diffuses from the endothelial cells toward the adjacent vascular smooth muscle cells, causing the muscle cells to relax. Under normal conditions there is a small but continuous release of NO from endothelial cells. The relaxing effect of NO antagonizes the contracting effect of the continuous sympathetic nerve stimulation described below. This exemplifies how the vasculature is under the constant influence of counteracting forces so that the final level of vascular resistance represents the balance of these influences.

The release of NO from endothelial cells helps maintain a constant velocity of blood flow. Up to this point we have only been concerned with how much blood is flowing (volume/time) and not how fast it is flowing (volume/distance). To increase the volume of blood flowing through a vessel in a given amount of time, the velocity at which it is flowing has to increase. Endothelial cells sense the velocity at which blood flows past their surface and act to keep this velocity constant by changing their release of NO. How they sense velocity is unknown. If the volume-flow of blood through a vessel increases, the associated increase in flow-velocity is sensed by the endothelial cells lining the vessel, which release more NO. The elevated NO relaxes the neighboring smooth muscle cells, decreasing resistance, and therefore both the volume and velocity of blood flow. In this way, the release of NO acts as a negative feedback system to maintain a constant velocity of blood flow. The opposite will happen when blood flow is reduced.

Autoregulation of Blood Flow

- Autoregulation is the maintenance of constant organ blood flow in the face of changing systemic arterial pressure.
- Autoregulation is greater in some organs than others.
- Autoregulation results from local changes in vascular resistance in response to changes in systemic arterial pressure.
- Two possible mechanisms are myogenic and metabolic.

Autoregulation is the ability of an organ to maintain a relatively constant blood flow in the face of changes in systemic arterial pressure. This relationship is illustrated in Figure 3–7. Several organs of the body exhibit autoregulation, including the brain, heart, kidneys, and skeletal muscle. However, not all organs exhibit the same level of autoregulation. Some organs, like the brain, are better able than other organs, like skeletal muscle, to maintain a constant blood flow when systemic arterial pressure changes.

The observation that blood flow to some organs changes little when systemic arterial pressure changes means that the arteriolar resistance of organs exhibiting

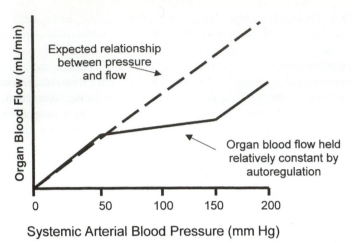

Figure 3–7
Blood flow through some organs remains constant even though systemic arterial pressure changes. This is known as autoregulation.

autoregulation is changing. To keep blood flow constant as systemic arterial pressure increases, arteriolar resistance must increase and as systemic arterial pressure decreases, resistance must decrease. In some way, the arterioles of organs exhibiting autoregulation sense the change in systemic arterial pressure and adjust their radius so that organ blood flow is held constant. There are two proposed hypotheses to explain autoregulation. The *metabolic hypothesis* states that autoregulation is chemically mediated. According to this hypothesis, as systemic arterial pressure increases, there is an increase in organ blood flow, which either washes away a vasodilator or washes in a vasoconstrictor. The net effect is that arteriolar resistance increases and blood flow is reduced. The opposite happens when systemic arterial pressure decreases. The *myogenic hypothesis* states that autoregulation is physically mediated. According to this hypothesis, as systemic arterial pressure increases, arterioles are stretched, causing the smooth muscle in the walls of the arterioles to contract. This contraction increases arteriolar resistance and reduces organ blood flow. The opposite happens when systemic arterial pressure decreases.

Control of Arterial Resistance

Global Control

- Sympathetic nerve activity is the primary global controller of resistance.
- Sympathetic nerves are tonically active, producing a background level of arteriolar resistance.

Global control of vascular resistance is achieved primarily by the sympathetic nervous system. Sympathetic nerves innervate smooth muscle cells of the arterioles and when they release their neurotransmitter norepinephrine, the smooth muscle cells contract, causing resistance to increase. Norepinephrine released from sympathetic nerve endings acts on *alpha-1 adrenergic receptors* on vascular smooth muscle cells increasing intracellular Ca concentration and inducing contraction.

Under normal conditions, sympathetic nerves are continuously active so the resistance of the arterioles is slightly elevated. This is good for two reasons. First, because of this elevated resistance, local chemicals can produce a decrease in resistance as occurs during active hyperemia or with the release of NO. In this way, constant sympathetic nerve activity enables local control of vascular resistance. Second, a decrease in sympathetic nerve activity produces a decrease in resistance because the smooth muscle cells are not being stimulated as much. Since sympathetic nerves innervate arterioles throughout the body, a decrease in sympathetic nerve activity will simultaneously lower resistance throughout the body. So, without the background level of sympathetic nerve activity, vascular resistance would not be able to be reduced.

Competition Between Local and Global Control

- Goal of local control of arteriolar resistance is to maintain adequate blood flow to meet the metabolic demands of an organ.
- Goal of global control of arteriolar resistance is to maintain an adequate systemic arterial pressure so that the brain and heart receive adequate blood flow.
- Competition between these goals can arise.

Competition between local and global control of arteriolar resistance can develop in association with many normal and abnormal situations. The sequence of events that occurs during a severe blood loss (hemorrhage) illustrates this competition. The reduction in blood volume causes the systemic arterial pressure to fall and initiates a reflex increase in sympathetic nerve activity (to be discussed in a subsequent section). This increases the resistance of arterioles in most organs of the body. The elevated resistance does two things. First, it helps to raise systemic arterial pressure toward normal by minimizing the amount of blood flowing to specific organs, which in turn augments the amount available to perfuse the brain and heart. Second, because of the reduced organ blood flow, flow and metabolic demand are no longer in balance and local chemicals that relax arteriolar smooth muscle cells accumulate. If blood volume is not restored soon enough, local factors counteract the effect of sympathetic nerve stimulation and arteriolar resistance is reduced, blood pressure falls, and the brain and heart do not receive adequate blood flow.

ROLE OF VENOUS SYSTEM IN MAINTAINING BLOOD PRESSURE

Characteristics of the Venous System

- Serves the role of a blood reservoir
- Compliant, that is, volume change produces little pressure change
- Compliance influenced by sympathetic nerve activity

The venous side of the systemic vasculature contains approximately two thirds of the total blood volume, yet the pressure within the venous system is less than that in the arterial system. The reason for this is that venous vessels are more *compliant* than arterial vessels. This means that veins can contain a larger volume of blood at a lower pressure. The low compliance of the venous system arises from the fact that the walls of the veins contain fewer smooth muscle cells and connective material as comparable arteries of the same diameter. This makes the veins less stiff and easier to expand. The consequence of this high compliance is that increases or decreases in cardiac output do not produce large changes in venous pressure. Therefore, a high pressure-gradient can be maintained between the venous and arterial sides of the circulation.

However, the compliance of the venous system can be altered through sympathetic nerve stimulation. Just as in the arterial circulation, there is a continuous level of sympathetic nerve activity, which means that the smooth muscle cells within the vessel wall are always slightly contracted and contributing to the stiffness of the wall. An increase in sympathetic nerve activity will further stimulate the venous smooth muscle cells through *alpha-1 receptors,* decreasing the compliance of the veins. A decrease in sympathetic nerve stimulation will reduce the stimulation of venous smooth muscle cells and they will relax, increasing the compliance.

Impact of Venous Return

- The volume of blood returning to the ventricles through the veins (venous return) influences cardiac output—a direct relationship between venous return and cardiac output.
- There is a direct relationship between blood volume and the magnitude of venous return.
- There is a direct relationship between the level of sympathetic nerve activity and venous return.

The volume of blood returning to the right ventricle determines end diastolic volume, that is, preload. The greater this volume (the greater the venous return), the greater will be the preload and therefore the greater will be the cardiac output of the right ventricle. Since the right and left ventricles are in series, an increase in right ventricular cardiac output will result in an increase in left ventricular cardiac output. In a similar manner, a decrease in venous return will result in a decrease in cardiac output. Therefore, changes in venous return, through its effect on cardiac output, will produce changes in arterial blood pressure.

Changes in blood volume influence the magnitude of venous return and therefore cardiac output. Even though the veins are compliant, a decrease in venous volume will still cause a decrease in venous pressure. This means that venous return and cardiac output will be decreased. The opposite occurs following an increase in blood volume.

An increase in sympathetic nerve activity will decrease venous compliance and increase venous return and cardiac output. A decrease in venous compliance means that the veins hold less blood at a given pressure. When compliance decreases due to increased sympathetic nerve activity, this excess blood volume is displaced toward the heart, increasing venous return and cardiac output. The opposite occurs with a decrease in sympathetic nerve activity. Therefore, sympathetic nerve activity influences arterial blood pressure by changing venous compliance, producing a change in venous return and cardiac output.

NUTRIENT AND FLUID EXCHANGE ACROSS THE CAPILLARY WALL

General Properties

> - Capillary wall is the site for exchange of substances between blood and cells of the body.
> - Capillary wall is permeable to small molecules except in the brain.
> - Movement of substances across the capillary wall occurs by diffusion.

Unlike other portions of the vasculature, the capillary wall is permeable to most substances. This is because the capillary wall is composed of a single layer of endothelial cells that have porous intercellular connections. There are some important exceptions to this statement. Large molecules like the protein albumin are unable to cross the capillary wall. Because large molecules are trapped in the vascular compartment while water can freely move across the capillary wall, the impermeable molecules will produce an osmotic pressure. Also, capillaries in the brain are not very permeable, greatly limiting the movement of molecules between the brain and blood. This impermeability creates the *blood-brain barrier*. Only in four discrete areas in or near the base of the brain are there areas of increased permeability where exchange occurs. Aside from these exceptions, the capillaries are the site for exchange of substances between the blood and the cells of the body.

The movement of substances between the blood and cells occurs solely by diffusion. Therefore, the direction of movement depends on whether the concentration gradient favors movement into the blood or toward the cells.

Capillary Osmotic Pressure

- Water freely moves across the capillary wall.
- Large protein molecules like albumin in the blood cannot cross the capillary wall.
- Albumin produces an osmotic pressure drawing water into the blood.

Because water, but not large protein molecules, crosses the capillary wall easily, blood proteins generate an osmotic pressure. Large proteins such as albumin are present in blood but not in the spaces around the cells of the body *(interstitial space)*. Therefore, the concentration gradient favors their movement out of the blood. However, they cannot cross the capillary wall. This concentration imbalance means that water is drawn into the blood to dilute the protein and make its concentration equal to that in the interstitial space. Therefore, blood proteins are osmotic particles that produce an osmotic pressure. The magnitude of this osmotic pressure equals about 25 mm Hg. If this force is not opposed, water will continue to move from the cells through the interstitial space and into the blood. However, the osmotic pressure generated by the blood proteins is opposed by the capillary blood pressure.

Blood Pressure Opposes Capillary Osmotic Pressure

- Capillary blood pressure forces water out of the capillary.
- Capillary blood pressure opposes the osmotic pressure produced by blood proteins.
- When capillary blood pressure is greater than osmotic pressure, filtration occurs; reabsorption occurs if the opposite is true.
- In lung capillaries only reabsorption occurs; in kidney capillaries only filtration occurs.

Because the capillary wall is leaky, the blood pressure forces water across the capillary wall like water out of a garden soaker hose. The walls of other vessels of the body are composed of multiple layers of cells and connective material so the blood pressure cannot drive fluid through the vessel wall. However, it does drive water across the capillary wall.

Over the length of a typical capillary in the body, the blood pressure declines from about 35 mm Hg to about 15 mm Hg due to the resistance of the capillary. This means that at the arterial end of the capillary, the force driving water out of the blood is greater than the force at the venous end of the capillary. As indicated above, the osmotic pressure due to blood proteins is approximately 25 mm Hg. Assuming osmotic pressure remains constant along the length of the capillary, blood pressure at the arterial end of the capillary is greater than the osmotic pressure, while at the venous end it is less. At the arterial end of the capillary, the balance between blood pressure and osmotic pressure favors the movement of water out of the capillary; at the venous end it favors movement of water into the capillary. Movement of water out of the capillary is called *filtration,* and the movement into the capillary is called *reabsorption.* The relationship between capillary blood pressure and osmotic pressure is diagramed in Figure 3–8.

In the capillary beds of the lungs and kidney, the balance between blood and osmotic pressures are such that only reabsorption or filtration occurs, respectively. The capillaries of the lung exhibit only reabsorption because pulmonary capillary pressure is normally less than capillary osmotic pressure so fluid is always drawn into the capillary blood. This is good because it keeps the alveoli of the lungs dry, maximizing the diffusion of gases between the blood and the air. Failure of the left ventricle causes lung capillary blood pressure to rise, producing filtration, lung edema, and difficult breathing. The capillaries of the kidney exhibit only filtration because renal capillary blood pressure is greater than capillary osmotic pressure. This is good because the filtered fluid passes through the tubules of the kidney where it is processed and adjustments are made to maintain a normal blood composition and volume.

Blood Pressure and Transcapillary Water Movement

- Increase in capillary blood pressure increases filtration.
- Decrease in capillary blood pressure increases reabsorption.
- Vascular resistance through its effect on capillary blood pressure alters transcapillary water movement.

Changes in systemic arterial or venous blood pressures cause changes in transcapillary water filtration or reabsorption. If everything else is unchanged, an increase in systemic arterial or venous blood pressures will increase transcapillary water filtration and decrease reabsorption because of the increase in capillary blood pressure. The opposite occurs when either blood pressure falls.

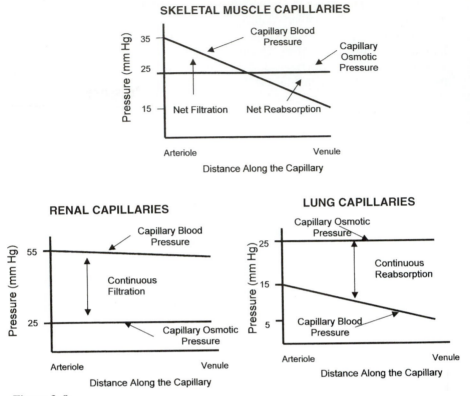

Figure 3–8
The relative magnitudes of capillary hydrostatic pressure and blood osmotic pressure determine the direction of fluid movement across capillary endothelia. These graphs plot hydrostatic and osmotic pressures as a function of capillary position for three different capillary beds in the body. In skeletal muscle both filtration and reabsorption occur, but in renal capillaries there is only filtration and in lung capillaries only reabsorption.

Changes in arteriolar and venular resistance produce opposite changes in capillary blood pressure and, therefore, opposite changes in filtration and reabsorption. Local changes in vascular resistance that may not alter systemic blood pressure produce local changes in capillary blood pressure. If resistance increases upstream from a capillary, capillary blood pressure decreases, while if resistance increases downstream from a capillary, capillary blood pressure increases. An increase in arteriolar resistance will produce a fall in blood pressure downstream from the site of resistance increase, that is, in the capillary. So, an increase in arteriolar resistance will lower capillary blood pressure, decrease filtration, and increase reabsorption. The opposite will happen if arteriolar resistance decreases. An increase in venular resistance will produce an increase in blood pressure upstream from the site of resistance increase, that is, in the capillary. So, an increase in venular resistance will increase capillary blood pressure, increase filtration, and decrease reabsorption. The opposite will happen if venular resistance decreases.

Transcapillary Water Movement and Blood Pressure

> • During times of low arterial blood pressure, reabsorption predominates, which increases blood volume and blood pressure.

A decrease in systemic arterial blood pressure directly lowers capillary blood pressure as well as initiates a homeostatic increase in arteriolar resistance, which also lowers capillary blood pressure. This reduction in capillary blood pressure favors reabsorption of water from the interstitial space, which helps to increase blood volume and bring blood pressure back to normal. In this way, water is drawn from the cells of the body through the interstitial space into the blood.

Transcapillary Water Movement and Edema

> • Excess filtration produces increased interstitial volume or edema.
> • Elevated capillary blood pressure produces edema.
> • Reduced blood osmotic pressure produces edema.

A sustained increase in capillary blood pressure causes water accumulation in the interstitial space, which is known as *edema*. If the pumping ability of either the left ventricle or the right ventricle is dramatically reduced, blood pressure rises upstream of the failing ventricle. If this is the left ventricle, then pressure in the veins leading from the lungs increases, which means that pulmonary capillary blood pressure increases. An elevation of pulmonary capillary blood pressure increases water filtration out of the blood into the interstitial space of the lungs causing pulmonary edema. The pulmonary edema decreases gas exchange in the lungs, which is sensed by the person as shortness of breath. If the right ventricle is failing, then pressure in the systemic veins increases causing an increase in systemic capillary blood pressure. Water filtration increases and accumulates in the interstitium of the legs and feet. This appears as swollen feet and ankles.

A decrease in blood osmotic pressure occurs with protein deficiency and produces edema. In severe malnutrition the concentration of albumin in the blood falls. Since albumin is the primary osmotic particle in blood, a decrease in albumin concentration lowers the blood's osmotic pressure. This means that capillary blood pressure exceeds the osmotic pressure of the blood for a longer distance along the capillary and so filtration exceeds reabsorption. This excess filtration and subsequent increase in interstitial water volume can appear as a swollen abdomen.

INTEGRATED CONTROL OF BLOOD PRESSURE

Pressure Receptors

- Pressure receptors or baroreceptors detect changes in intravascular pressure and volume by sensing vascular wall tension.
- Two classes of baroreceptors are high pressure and low pressure.
- High pressure baroreceptors are located in the aorta and carotid artery and monitor systemic arterial blood pressure.
- Degree of high pressure baroreceptor stimulation is directly related to magnitude and rate of change of blood pressure.
- Low pressure baroreceptors are located in large veins, pulmonary artery, and right atrium and monitor venous volume.
- Right atrium releases atrial natriuretic hormone, which causes renal salt and water excretion.

The body monitors blood pressure through stretch receptors *(baroreceptors)* located in the walls of specific blood vessels and the right atrium. Sensory nerve endings, located in the walls of these structures, are stretched when the vessel wall is expanded by an increase in intravascular pressure, and they send more action potentials to the brain. If pressure and wall stretch decrease, the number of action potentials sent to the brain decreases. Under normal levels of blood pressure and volume, these receptors are under some degree of stretch and so are continuously sending a constant number of action potentials to the brain.

There are two general classes of baroreceptors: high pressure and low pressure. *High-pressure baroreceptors* are located in the arch of the aorta as it leaves the left ventricle and in the two carotid arteries that lead to the brain. Because of their anatomical location, these receptors measure systemic arterial blood pressure, which is the highest pressure in the cardiovascular system. High-pressure baroreceptors respond not only to the absolute level of the blood pressure, but also to how rapidly it changes.

Low-pressure baroreceptors are located in the great veins leading into the right atrium, the pulmonary artery leaving the right ventricle, and the wall of the right atrium. Because these baroreceptors are located on the venous side of the circulation where pressure is low, they are called low-pressure receptors. In fact, because the compliance of these structures is low, small changes in pressure produce large changes in volume, and so the body interprets changes in the activity of the low-pressure baroreceptors as changes in blood volume. So, the low-pressure baroreceptors are sometimes called *volume receptors*.

The right atrium not only sends information about blood volume to the brain through sensory nerve fibers but it also releases a hormone, *atrial natriuretic hormone*, when the volume increases. This hormone acts on the kidney to stimulate excretion of salt and water, which acts to return blood volume toward normal.

Medullary Cardiovascular Center

* Cardiovascular center integrates sensory information about the status of the cardiovascular system and initiates adjustments to maintain an appropriate systemic arterial blood pressure.
* Cardiovascular center is a collection of neurons located in the medulla of the brain.

An essential component of any homeostatic system is an integration center. The *cardiovascular center* (CV center) is such an integration center. It is a collection of neurons in the medulla of the brain that receives sensory information from a variety of sources, compares this information with the set point for systemic arterial blood pressure, and initiates responses to maintain an appropriate blood pressure. This is the seat for central control of blood pressure.

The sensory input to the CV center is extensive. The primary peripheral receptors that monitor blood pressure are the low- and high-pressure baroreceptors. Sensory fibers from the baroreceptors go to the CV center. An increase in pressure stretches these receptors increasing the frequency of action potentials sent to the CV center, which initiate responses designed to lower blood pressure. The CV center also receives information from the *respiratory center*, a neighboring collection of nerves involved in controlling respiration. Generally, an increase in respiration rate leads to an increase in heart rate and blood pressure because of stimulation of the CV center by neurons from the respiratory center. The CV center also receives information from higher areas in the brain such as the hypothalamus, limbic system, and cerebral cortex. Input from these areas can override the homeostatic activity of the cardiovascular system. A familiar example of the influence of higher areas of the brain on the CV center is the change in blood pressure associated with extreme events in life. The changes in blood pressure can range from a rapid elevation associated with a threatening situation to a rapid fall leading to fainting associated with a very emotional situation.

Interrelationship Between Cardiovascular and Renal Systems

- Cardiovascular reflexes are designed for short-term regulation of blood pressure.
- Kidneys have a long-term effect on blood pressure through the control of salt and water balance.

Cardiovascular reflexes mediated through the high- and low-pressure baroreceptors regulate blood pressure over short periods of time (minutes to days). The cardiovascular reflexes are designed for rapid short-term corrections of blood pressure. Because reflex corrections are mediated primarily through the sympathetic nervous system, they are initiated rapidly. However, if blood pressure is chronically altered, baroreceptors adapt to this sustained change and no longer signal the cardiovascular center that pressure is abnormal.

    The kidneys through their ability to control the salt and water balance of the body also have a significant impact on the control of blood pressure. Regulating blood volume is critical for maintaining a constant blood pressure, and the kidneys do this through altering the excretion of salt and water. However, this effect occurs over hours to days. Therefore, the kidneys influence blood pressure over the long term.

EXAMPLES OF INTEGRATED CARDIOVASCULAR RESPONSES

Loss of Blood Volume

- Loss of blood volume produces a fall in systemic arterial blood pressure.
- Fall in blood pressure initiates a sympathetic nerve mediated compensatory response.
- Cardiovascular responses to reestablish normal blood pressure include:
  —Increased heart rate
  —Increased stroke volume
  —Increased arteriolar resistance
  —Increased transcapillary water reabsorption

The response of the cardiovascular system to a reduction in blood volume varies with the magnitude and duration of the loss. When you donate a unit (500 mL) of blood over a 15-min period, your body compensates so that blood pressure does not change, and the volume is replaced through the normal ingestion of fluids. However, larger volume losses require more direct intervention. Volume losses up to 30–40% of total blood volume can be tolerated if the loss is corrected within 30 min. A reduction in blood volume can be absolute, that is, a loss of blood from the vascular compartment to another body cavity or to the exterior of the body. However, there can also be a functional decrease in volume secondary to a massive decrease in arteriolar resistance (eg, emotional fainting) or increase in venous compliance.

A decrease in absolute or functional blood volume produces a fall in systemic arterial blood pressure, which reduces venous return, EDV, SV, and cardiac output. This is sensed by the high-pressure baroreceptors that decrease the rate at which they send action potentials to the medullar cardiovascular center. This causes the cardiovascular center to increase the activity of sympathetic nerves, which act on the heart and vasculature. In the absence of a functioning sympathetic nervous system, our ability to recover from a severe blood loss is cut in half, so the sympathetic nervous system is very important.

Increased sympathetic nerve activity to the heart elevates heart rate because the released norepinephrine increases the rate of spontaneous depolarization of SA node cells. The released norepinephrine also acts on ventricular muscle cells increasing their contractility and, therefore, force of contraction. This means that at any given end diastolic volume the stroke volume is elevated toward normal. The combination of an elevation in heart rate and stroke volume elevates cardiac output toward normal. Increasing cardiac output helps bring arterial pressure back toward normal.

Increased sympathetic nerve activity to the vasculature, via norepinephrine, causes constriction of arterioles increasing vascular resistance. This helps raise arterial blood pressure toward normal. In addition, venous smooth muscle will be stimulated to contract, which decreases venous compliance and displaces this additional blood volume to the heart. The added volume increases venous return, EDV, and cardiac output and helps raise arterial blood pressure.

The increased sympathetic nerve activity to the vasculature does not increase the arteriolar resistance in coronary or cerebral circulations. This is because these organs have strong autoregulatory responses. The fall in systemic arterial pressure produced by the loss of blood volume, produces an autoregulatory decrease in arteriolar resistance, which maintains adequate cerebral and coronary flows.

The elevation in arteriolar resistance in response to sympathetic nerve stimulation produces another beneficial effect in addition to raising systemic arterial pressure. Pressure is elevated upstream from the constricted arterioles (systemic arterial pressure) but the pressure downstream from the arterioles (capillary blood pressure) is reduced. The fall in capillary blood pressure means that the force driving water from the capillaries is reduced enabling more water to be drawn into capillary blood by the osmotic pressure of the blood. This causes filtration to be reduced and water reabsorption to be increased. The increased reabsorption helps return blood volume to normal.

Involvement of Other Systems

- Kidneys decrease urine output.
- Angiotensin II and aldosterone are released.
- There is an increased sense of thirst.

Other organ systems become involved to reduce water loss. The role of the kidneys in volume control is discussed in detail in chapter 4, however, in general urine output is reduced and the kidney stimulates the formation of the hormone angiotensin II. *Angiotensin II* acts on arteriolar smooth muscle cells to cause contraction and helps raise resistance. In addition, it stimulates the secretion of *aldosterone* from the adrenal cortex. This hormone stimulates the kidney to reabsorb sodium chloride, which helps hold water in the vascular compartment. Also, nerve activity from the cardiovascular center stimulates the hypothalamus to release *antidiuretic hormone (ADH or vasopressin).* ADH stimulates arterioles to constrict increasing resistance, and it stimulates water reabsorption by the kidney.

   All of these reflex responses try to compensate for the fall in blood volume but they cannot replace the volume that is lost from the body. To do this, the sense of thirst is stimulated. This is initiated in part by the cardiovascular center. The cardiovascular center sends information to higher centers in the brain, which generate a desire for water intake. Finally, the elevated blood levels of angiotensin II stimulate thirst by stimulating higher brain centers.

Cardiovascular Changes Induced Upon Standing

- Moving from the prone to the erect position causes blood to be distributed to the legs, which decreases ventricular filling and cardiac output just like with a loss of blood volume.
- Reflex cardiovascular responses are similar to those caused by a loss of blood volume.

When you move from the prone to the erect position, blood pools in the veins of your legs reducing venous return, cardiac output, and blood pressure. In the standing position, the vessels in the legs are like columns of liquid. The weight of this liquid column distends the walls of the vessels. The veins, being more compliant than the arteries, expand more and fill with blood. This reduces the amount of blood that can flow back to the heart, reducing cardiac output and blood pressure. The cardiovascular response to this fall in pressure is identical to that of a loss of blood volume, that is, an increase in sympathetic nerve activity.

Because a change in position produces a small change in blood pressure, it takes the reflexes no longer than 1 minute to bring the blood pressure to normal. Relative to the prone position, the heart rate and arteriolar resistance will be slightly elevated indicating the presence of the elevated sympathetic nerve activity.

Cardiovascular Response to Prolonged Standing

- With prolonged standing, capillary blood pressure increases in the legs increasing filtration and reducing blood volume.
- Contraction of skeletal muscle helps pump blood toward the heart reducing capillary blood pressure and filtration.

When moving from the prone to the erect position, both venous and arterial pressures in the dependent leg vessels increase due to the weight of the blood column. Venous pressure can increase to over 80 mm Hg. This increase in venous pressure causes an increase in capillary blood pressure and filtration of fluid out of the capillary blood. With prolonged standing, the elevated filtration can lead to reduced blood volume. In addition, the effect of sympathetic nerve stimulation alone is inadequate to maintain a normal blood pressure if standing is prolonged. However, if the individual moves or contracts leg muscles, the contracting skeletal muscles act as a pump forcing blood out of the veins toward the heart. This pumping effect is made possible by the presence of venous valves. As the skeletal muscles contract, blood within the veins is forced past the valves and when the muscles relax, the blood is prevented from flowing back because the valve closes. In this way, contraction of skeletal muscles moves venous blood toward the heart and decreases venous pressure.

RENAL PHYSIOLOGY

·

GENERAL PRINCIPLES
Kidney Functions

- Kidneys regulate water and electrolyte levels.
- Kidneys regulate acid-base balance.
- Kidneys excrete metabolic waste products and foreign substances.
- Hormones produced are angiotensin II, 1,25-dihydroxyvitamin D_3, and erythropoietin.

The kidney is a key organ in the maintenance of homeostasis. Through its excretion of water and electrolytes, the kidney controls cell volume and the blood levels of many important ions that influence membrane excitability. As discussed in the cardiovascular chapter, the kidney has a long-term impact on blood pressure because of its role in volume control. The kidney along with the lungs regulates the hydrogen ion concentration of the blood keeping it within very narrow limits. The blood levels of metabolic waste products such as urea, uric acid, creatinine, and bilirubin are prevented from rising to toxic levels by the kidney. Finally, the kidney is involved in the production of several important hormones. The kidney initiates the synthesis of the hormone angiotensin II, which is important in regulating blood pressure and aldosterone secretion from the adrenal cortex. The kidney synthesizes the active form of vitamin D (1,25-dihydroxyvitamin D_3) needed for proper Ca metabolism and the hormone erythropoietin, which stimulates red blood cell formation by bone marrow. It can be seen that the kidney has an impact on a multitude of organs and body functions.

Basic Kidney Structure

- The nephron is the basic subunit of the kidney.
- Renal arterioles lead to glomerular capillary tufts, which are the site of blood filtration.
- Bowman's capsule receives this filtrate, which is modified as it passes along the kidney tubules.
- A single kidney tubule is divided into four major sequential sections: proximal tubule, loop of Henle, distal tubule, and collecting duct, each with unique characteristics.
- Capillaries surround kidney tubules enabling exchange between blood and tubular fluid.

The *nephron* is the basic subunit of the kidney. It is composed of two components: the glomerulus and the renal tubule.

The renal arteries to the left and right kidneys originate directly from the abdominal aorta and begin to branch a short distance after they enter each kidney. After repeated branching a large number of arterioles (approximately 1 million) end in capillary tufts, the majority of which are in the outer third or cortex of the kidney. Each capillary tuft is called a *glomerulus*. Unlike other vascular beds, the vessel leaving the glomerulus is an arteriole rather than a venule. The significance of this will become apparent when we examine control of kidney function. Surrounding each glomerulus is a hollow capsule called *Bowman's capsule*. The relationship between these two structures can be visualized as a fist (glomerulus) pushed into an inflated balloon (Bowman's capsule). This means there are two cell layers, the capillary endothelium of the glomerulus and the epithelial cells of Bowman's capsule, separating these two structures.

Between these cell layers is a basement membrane composed primarily of glycoproteins and mucopolysaccharides. The endothelium of the glomerulus is porous because of spaces between the cells. The epithelial cells of Bowman's capsule are called *podocytes* and look like a layer of octopi with their arms interdigitating. This also makes the podocytes porous. Because of the porous nature of these layers, some of the blood flowing through the capillaries is forced across the capillary endothelium, through the basement membrane, and between the arms of the podocytes. These layers act as screens preventing substances as large proteins and red blood cells from passing through. However, water, ions, hormones, and other small molecules pass easily into Bowman's capsule. This fluid is called an *ultrafiltrate of blood*. About 125 mL of ultrafiltrate are formed each minute from the over 600 mL of blood that flows through the kidney every minute.

Bowman's capsule is the beginning of the *renal tubule* in which the fluid forced into Bowman's capsule from the glomerulus is processed as it becomes urine and collects in the bladder. The renal tubule is divided into four sections: *proximal tubule, loop of Henle, distal tubule* and *collecting duct.* The proximal tubule as it leaves Bowman's capsule remains in the cortical layer of the kidney. When it becomes the loop of Henle, the first portion of the loop dives into the interior or medulla of the kidney before turning upward again into the cortex where it becomes the distal tubule. Distal tubules from many renal tubules come together to form the collecting duct, which extends from the cortex back through the medulla. Many collecting ducts combine and empty into the calyx of the renal pelvis. The pelvis is continuous with the *ureter,* the tube carrying the fluid to the bladder. Each of these segments has unique structural and functional characteristics, which will be examined later. In addition, we will see that the structure and anatomical relationship of the loop of Henle and the collecting duct enable the kidney to adjust both the volume and osmolarity of the urine.

As indicated above, the vessel leaving the glomerulus is an arteriole. It then branches into a second capillary network called the *peritubular capillaries.* These capillaries surround specific segments of the tubule, and they return water and substances reabsorbed by the tubule to the general circulation, as well as deliver needed nutrients to the tubule. The peritubular capillaries empty into venules, which continue to coalesce to form the renal vein. The renal vein leaves the kidney near where the renal artery entered the kidney.

Basic Renal Terminology

- Glomerular filtration rate is the amount of fluid moving into Bowman's capsule per unit time.
- Renal blood flow is the amount of blood flowing through the kidney per unit of time.
- Filtration is the process by which substances enter Bowman's capsule.
- Reabsorption is the process by which substances move from inside to outside the tubule.
- Secretion is the process by which substances move from outside to inside the tubule.
- Excretion refers to substances that pass from the kidney into the bladder.

A few terms used in renal physiology need to be defined. *Glomerular filtration rate (GFR)* is the amount of fluid that passes from the glomerulus into Bowman's capsule per unit of time. Because of the way in which it is determined, GFR represents the average rate of all 1 million glomeruli. *Renal blood flow (RBF)* refers to the amount of blood that flows through the kidney per unit of time. Like GFR, RBF also represents an average.

Four terms are used to describe movement of substances into and out of the renal tubule. When a substance enters the tubule from the glomerular capillary bed, it is said to be *filtrated*. Substances can also enter by passing across the wall of any segment of the tubule. This is called *secretion*. Once within the lumen of the tubule, a substance can leave by passing across the wall, which is called *reabsorption*. Or, it can leave in the urine, called *excretion*. In a general sense, a substance can move in and out of the tubule by one or more of these processes depending upon where along the length of the tubule it is and the needs of the body at that moment. However, it is the ability of the kidney to selectively move specific substances into and out of the tubule in a very controlled and coordinated manner that makes normal kidney function so critical to life.

CLEARANCE

Clearance Used to Measure GFR and RPF

- Clearance is based on the principle of conservation of mass.
- Clearance is the volume of blood per unit of time that had all of a particular substance removed by the kidney.
- The clearance formula is $C_X = (V_U \times [X]_U)/[X]_P$.
- The clearance of substances with specific properties enables one to determine GFR and RPF.

Glomerular filtration rate and renal blood flow are two values that are important for assessing kidney function. But they are not measured easily by any direct method. Therefore, an indirect method is used that relies on the conservation of mass.

Let's assume that a substance, X, is present in the blood at a concentration of 1 g/mL (see Figure 4–1). As the blood flows through the glomeruli, a portion is filtered and the remainder flows out of the glomerular capillary bed. Because of filtration, some of X is carried into Bowman's capsule. If X can pass freely into Bowman's capsule, then its concentration in the fluid in Bowman's capsule will equal that in the capillary blood. The rate (g/min) at which X appears in Bowman's capsule will equal the rate at which fluid flows into the capsule (GFR, mL/min) times the concentration of X in the blood (g/mL). Assuming GFR equals 125 mL/min then the rate at which X enters the kidney can be calculated as follows:

$$\text{Rate of X IN} = \text{GFR} \times [X]_P = 125 \text{ mL/min} \times 1 \text{ g/mL} = 125 \text{ g/min}$$

Assuming that once in the renal tubule, X cannot cross the tubule wall, the amount leaving in the urine per minute must equal the amount entering the tubule

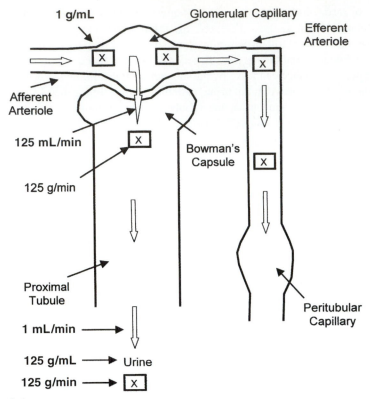

Figure 4–1
This figure illustrates the principle of clearance and how it can be used to determine glomerular filtration rate.

per minute. The rate at which X leaves the kidney is the urine flow rate (mL/min) times the urine concentration of X (g/mL). If the urine flow rate is 1 mL/min and the concentration of X in the urine is determined to be 125 g/mL, then:

$$\text{Rate of X OUT} = V_U \times [X]_U = 1 \text{ mL/min} \times 125 \text{ g/mL} = 125 \text{ g/min}$$

As calculated, in 1 minute, 125 g of X appeared in the urine. Since the concentration of X in blood is 1 g/mL, then in 1 minute, 125 mL of blood must have given up its quantity of X. That is, 125 mL of blood were "cleared" of X. Or, stated another way, the clearance of X is 125 mL/min.

In this example, the clearance of X, 125 mL/min, equals the GFR. This is not coincidental but due to the special properties of X, freely filtered and neither reabsorbed nor secreted. Because of these properties the Rate of X IN = Rate of X OUT and therefore:

$$GFR \times [X]_P = V_U \times [X]_U.$$

Or solving for GFR:

$$GFR = (V_U \times [X]_U)/[X]_P.$$

If there was a substance with properties similar to those of X, then GFR could be calculated. There is a naturally occurring substance, *creatinine*, that is normally present in the blood and is not reabsorbed and minimally secreted by the kidney. By measuring urine flow rate and the concentration of creatinine in the blood and urine, the GFR can be calculated. Because of the characteristics of creatinine, you can say that the clearance of creatinine is the GFR.

The equation for GFR represents a special case for a substance with properties like creatinine but can be generalized for any substance X in which case it becomes the clearance equation:

$$C_X = (V_U \times [X]_U)/[X]_P.$$

The clearance of any substance in the blood (eg, Na, K, or glucose) can be calculated using this equation. In most cases clearance is very small since most of what is filtered into Bowman's capsule is returned to the blood by the time the fluid has passed along the tubule and reaches the end of the collecting duct.

The clearance equation can also be used to calculate *renal plasma flow (RPF)* if a substance with an additional property is used. This additional property is that all of it needs to be removed from the blood by the kidney through a combination of filtration and secretion. There is no substance naturally present in the body that meets this criterion, but a polysaccharide called para-aminohippuric acid (PAH) does. If PAH is infused so that its concentration in blood is low, the renal tubules can secrete any PAH that escapes filtration. This means that through filtration and secretion all of the PAH present in the blood is removed. This means that the blood is completely cleared of PAH and, therefore, the PAH clearance equals the RPF.

Renal blood flow can be derived from the calculation of RPF by taking into account the added volume occupied by the red blood cells. Red blood cell volume is the hematocrit (Hct), which is about 45%. Therefore,

$$RBF = RPF/(1 - Hct).$$

DETERMINANTS AND REGULATION OF GFR AND RPF

Determinants of GFR

- GFR is determined by five factors: filtration coefficient, capillary hydrostatic pressure, capillary osmotic pressure, Bowman's capsule hydrostatic pressure, Bowman's capsule osmotic pressure.
- $GFR = K_f \times [(P_{GC} + \Pi_{BC}) - (P_{BC} + \Pi_{GC})$.

GFR is determined by the balance of forces acting across the walls of the glomerulus and Bowman's capsule and the permeability property of the cells of these structures. The forces that drive fluid out of the glomerulus are the capillary blood pressure (P_{GC}) and the osmotic pressure (Π_{BC}) of the fluid in Bowman's capsule. The forces driving fluid into the glomerulus are the hydrostatic pressure (P_{BC}) of the fluid in Bowman's capsule and the osmotic pressure (Π_{GC}) of the blood within the glomerulus. The difference between these four forces determines the *net filtration pressure*, which is approximately 15 mm Hg.

$$\text{Net filtration pressure} = (P_{GC} + \Pi_{BC}) - (P_{BC} + \Pi_{GC})$$
$$= (55 + 0) - (15 + 25) = 15 \text{ mm Hg.}$$

Notice in this expression that the osmotic pressure of the fluid in Bowman's capsule (Π_{BC}) is zero. This is because the fluid that is filtered through the walls of the glomerular capillaries and Bowman's capsule is essentially free of proteins but contains the same concentration of ions (and other small molecules) as the blood. These particles do not exert an osmotic pressure because they can freely move into and out of Bowman's capsule. Therefore, the ultrafiltrate exerts little if any osmotic pressure to draw water into Bowman's capsule.

These physical forces would be of no consequence if the endothelial and epithelial cells that formed the glomerulus and Bowman's capsule, respectively, were impermeable. However, they are permeable and this permeability is reflected in a factor called the *filtration coefficient* (K_f). Therefore, the complete expression for GFR is

$$GFR = K_f \times [(P_{GC} + \Pi_{BC}) - (P_{BC} + \Pi_{GC})].$$

Regulation of GFR

> Changes in systemic arterial pressure, the radius of the renal arterioles, and the filtration coefficient normally regulate GFR.

Of the factors that determine GFR, the body normally alters some, while others change primarily during abnormal conditions. Those altered normally include systemic arterial pressure, renal arteriolar resistance, and filtration coefficient.

If systemic arterial pressure increases, then the pressure in the glomerular capillaries will increase and GFR will increase. The opposite will happen if systemic arterial pressure decreases.

As was described earlier, the glomerular capillary bed originates from an arteriole called the *afferent arteriole*, but ends in a second arteriole, the *efferent*

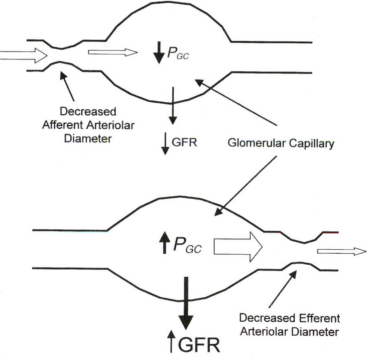

Figure 4–2
Changes in arteriolar resistance before (afferent) and after (efferent) the glomerular capillary bed have different effects on capillary hydrostatic pressure (P_{GC}) and therefore on glomerular filtration rate (GFR).

arteriole. Like arterioles elsewhere in the body their diameter can be altered by the action of nerves and hormones on the smooth muscle cells that exist in the walls of the arterioles. However, GFR is changed in opposite directions by changes in the diameter of afferent and efferent arterioles. As diagrammed in Figure 4–2, a decrease in the diameter of the afferent arteriole will cause a decrease in the glomerular capillary blood pressure and, therefore, in GFR. If the resistance of the arteriole leading into the glomerular capillary increases, pressure downstream of the resistance (P_{GC}) falls. The opposite will occur if the afferent arteriolar diameter increases (resistance decreases). However, if the efferent arteriolar diameter decreases, then the pressure upstream of the resistance change (P_{GC}) will increase and so will GFR. The opposite will happen if the diameter increases (resistance decreases).

The filtration coefficient can be altered by the contractile activity of an additional set of cells located among the podocytes. These cells are called *mesangial cells*. These cells can be stimulated to contract, and when this occurs they decrease the area available for filtration and thus decrease the filtration coefficient and GFR.

Under abnormal conditions changes can occur in plasma protein concentration and in the hydrostatic pressure within Bowman's capsule. During severe starvation or following severe burns over large areas of the body, the concentration of protein in the blood falls. This lowers the osmotic pressure of the blood (Π_{GC}) increasing the net filtration pressure and GFR. Bowman's capsule hydrostatic pressure (P_{BC}) can increase if the ureter becomes blocked such as with renal stones. This causes fluid to accumulate in the renal tubules, which backs up into Bowman's capsule and raises the hydrostatic pressure. This reduces the net filtration pressure and GFR.

Determinants and Regulation of RBF

- RBF is determined by systemic arterial blood pressure and renal vascular resistance.
- RBF demonstrates autoregulation.
- Autoregulation involves afferent not efferent arterioles.
- Autoregulation is explained either by the myogenic hypothesis or tubuloglomerular feedback.

Renal blood flow is determined by the systemic arterial blood pressure with increases resulting in an increase in RBF. A decrease produces the opposite effect. Also, changes in renal vascular resistance alter RBF with an increase in resistance decreasing flow and a decrease in resistance increasing flow.

Interestingly, over a range of systemic arterial blood pressures that occur normally, RBF does not increase as much as would be expected if the two were directly related. This relationship is illustrated in Figure 4–3. As can be seen in the figure, over a range of systemic arterial pressures, RBF remains fairly constant. For flow to remain constant as pressure increases implies that renal vascular resistance must be increasing. The tendency for blood flow to remain constant in the face of changing pressure is called *autoregulation*. The cerebral and coronary circulations also exhibit autoregulation. Notice in the figure that GFR changes in a similar way as RBF. This implies that the resistance change that maintains a constant RBF must involve the afferent arterioles, not the efferent arterioles. If the efferent arterioles were involved, then GFR would change as efferent resistance changed to maintain a constant RBF.

There are two hypotheses that describe renal vascular autoregulation: myogenic and tubuloglomerular feedback. According to the *myogenic hypothesis*, when systemic arterial pressure increases RBF, the afferent arterioles are stretched. This stretch stimulates them to contract increasing their resistance and maintaining a constant RBF. If RBF decreased, then the opposite would occur.

Tubuloglomerular feedback involves an interaction between the distal tubules and the afferent arterioles. The beginning portion of the distal tubule passes close to the afferent arteriole, and together they form a specialized structure called the *juxtaglomerular apparatus*. Specialized epithelial cells in this portion of the distal tubule, called *macula densa cells,* sense the amount of NaCl in the tubular fluid. With an increase in RBF there will be an increase in GFR, an increase in filtration, and an increase in the amount of NaCl passing by

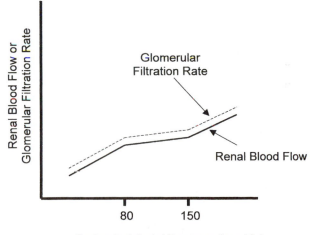

Figure 4–3
The kidney maintains a constant blood flow (autoregulation) and glomerular filtration rate over the physiological range of systemic arterial pressures.

the macula densa cells. In response to this increased NaCl, a yet unidentified substance is released that causes afferent arteriolar constriction. This constriction reduces RBF, GFR, and the amount of NaCl delivered to the macula densa cells. If RBF were to decrease, then the opposite would occur.

Interaction Between RBF and GFR

> With a large increase in efferent arteriolar resistance, GFR does not increase as much as expected because of an increase in glomerular capillary osmotic pressure produced by a decrease in RBF.

As discussed above, an increase in efferent arteriolar resistance produces opposite effects on RBF and GFR. RBF decreases and GFR increases. Under normal situations, blood leaving the glomerular capillary bed is at a higher osmotic pressure (Π_{GC}) than the blood entering because of the fluid lost as the ultrafiltrate. This rise in Π_{GC} is not sufficient to significantly limit GFR. However, with a large increase in efferent resistance, RBF is reduced enabling Π_{GC} to increase to such an extent that GFR is reduced. Therefore, GFR does not increase as much as expected with an increase in efferent arteriolar resistance because of the relationship between GFR, RBF, and Π_{GC}.

CHARACTERISTICS OF INDIVIDUAL NEPHRON SEGMENTS

Overview of Tubule Properties

> - Permeability properties of the luminal and basolateral membranes of the epithelial cells lining renal tubules are different, enabling directional movement of salt and water.
> - Proximal tubule reabsorbs isotonically a constant 60% of the GFR.
> - Loop of Henle reabsorbs more salt than water.
> - Distal tubule continues to reabsorb more salt than water.
> - Permeability of the collecting duct to salt and water is hormonally controlled by antidiuretic hormone and aldosterone.

The luminal and basolateral sides of the epithelial cells that line the renal tubules have different permeability properties. This difference in permeability is due to the existence of different transport proteins in the membranes of these two sides of the cell. This cellular polarity is crucial for directional movement of substances across the epithelial cell.

The epithelium of the proximal tubule is permeable
absorbs a constant 60% of the GFR. Reabsorption of wa
sorption of NaCl and an osmotic gradient between th
peritubular capillary blood.

The two limbs of the loop of Henle are not equally
water. The descending limb is permeable to water while
permeable to salt. The net effect is that more salt than wate

The distal tubule is minimally permeable to water a   ... salt than
water is reabsorbed. Because distal tubule fluid is dilute relative to blood, this
tubule is called the *diluting tubule.*

Two hormones, antidiuretic hormone and aldosterone, control the permeability of the collecting duct to salt and water. In the absence of these hormones,
little salt or water is reabsorbed and a large volume, dilute urine is produced. In
the presence of these hormones, salt and water reabsorption are high, and a low
volume, concentrated urine is formed.

Proximal Tubule Reabsorption of Salt and Water

- NaCl reabsorption is dependent upon the coordinated action of the Na-
  K-ATPase on the basolateral membrane of the epithelial cell and several
  facilitated transport systems on the luminal membrane of the epithelial
  cell.
- Water reabsorption follows and is dependent upon Na ion reabsorption.
- Water reabsorption is assisted by the elevated osmolarity of the peritubular capillary blood.

Na ions move from the tubular fluid into the proximal tubule epithelial cells because of a concentration gradient created by the Na-K-ATPase located in the
basolateral membrane of the cell. This is diagrammed in Figure 4–4. The Na-K-
ATPase moves Na^+ against a concentration gradient from inside to outside the
cell, which keeps the intracellular Na ion concentration low. The low intracellular Na ion concentration enables Na^+ in the tubular fluid to diffuse down this
concentration gradient causing reabsorption. The movement of Na^+ into the epithelial cells is coupled to the movement of other molecules into the cell as
shown in Figure 4–4. Because of this, the reabsorption of substances like amino
acids and glucose depend upon Na^+ reabsorption and ultimately upon the activity
of the Na-K-ATPase.

The fluid that enters the proximal tubule from Bowman's capsule exerts the
same osmotic pressure as the interstitial fluid. Its osmotic pressure is due to the
large number of Na ions present in the fluid. As Na^+ is reabsorbed by the epithelial cells, the osmotic pressure of the tubular fluid decreases. This means that

TUBULAR FLUID

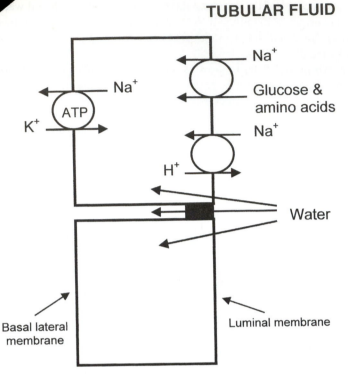

Figure 4–4

The major mechanisms by which molecules move across the epithelium of the proximal tubule are diagramed in this figure.

there is a gradient for water movement from the tubular fluid into the interstitial space. Water moves easily across the epithelial cells in response to this osmotic gradient. Therefore, water reabsorption follows Na⁺ reabsorption. If Na⁺ reabsorption is reduced, the reabsorption of water will be also. Some diuretics interfere with Na⁺ reabsorption in the proximal tubule and by this mechanism reduce water reabsorption.

The movement of water from the interstitial space into the blood is facilitated by the elevated osmotic pressure of the peritubular capillary blood. Remember that when some of the blood was filtered at the glomerulus, protein was left behind raising the osmotic pressure of the blood leaving the glomerulus. This blood next passes through the peritubular capillaries surrounding the proximal tubules. Because of this elevated osmotic pressure, water will be drawn from the interstitial space into the peritubular capillary blood completing water reabsorption.

Proximal Tubule Reabsorption of Glucose and Amino Acids

- Reabsorption of glucose and amino acids is coupled to the reabsorption of Na ions.
- Glucose reabsorption is overwhelmed when blood glucose is very high (diabetes).

As indicated in the previous section, the reabsorption of glucose and amino acids from the tubular fluid is linked to the reabsorption of Na ions. The structure of transport molecules located in the luminal membrane of the epithelial cells enable these proteins to simultaneously carry into the cell a Na ion and either a molecule of glucose or amino acid. The movement of glucose or amino acids into the cell is against a concentration gradient, but energy for this movement is provided by the downhill movement of Na^+ into the cell. This is an example of secondary active transport (see chapter 2).

The transport molecules for glucose are distinct from those that move amino acids, and classes of amino acids (neutral, acid, basic) have their own specific transport molecules. Generally, the concentration of glucose (5 mM) and amino acids (2 mM) are very low in the tubular fluid and, therefore, there are plenty of Na ions (140 mM) to permit complete reabsorption of glucose and amino acids by the end of the proximal tubule. However, in diabetes mellitus the blood glucose concentration can become so high that all the Na-glucose transport molecules are occupied (saturated) and some of the glucose escapes reabsorption. When this occurs, glucose is found in the urine.

Proximal Tubule Reabsorption of Bicarbonate Ions

- Bicarbonate reabsorption requires Na-dependent H ion secretion.
- Bicarbonate reabsorption occurs indirectly through the formation of CO_2 and H_2O.

The secretion of H ions from the proximal tubule epithelial cells occurs through a carrier mediated exchange process for Na ions (see Figure 4–5). Again, the movement of Na ions down their concentration gradient into epithelial cells is coupled though a carrier protein that moves H ions out of the epithelial cell (an example of counter-transport). These H ions do not acidify the tubular fluid but rather combine with the bicarbonate ions that are filtered into Bowman's capsule from the blood. The resulting carbonic acid rapidly dissociates into CO_2 and H_2O because of the action of the enzyme carbonic anhydrase located on the surface of the epithelial cells. The CO_2 diffuses into the epithelial cell where it recombines

TUBULAR FLUID

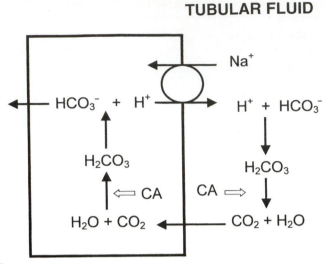

Figure 4–5
Reabsorption of bicarbonate ions in the proximal tubule requires the formation and break-down of carbonic acid (H_2CO_3) within the tubular fluid and epithelial cells. The enzyme carbonic anhydrase (CA) is essential for this process to occur.

with H_2O under the influence of cellular carbonic anhydrase to form carbonic acid. Carbonic acid once again dissociates into H and bicarbonate ions. The H ions are secreted again in exchange for Na ions and the bicarbonate ions diffuse across the basal lateral side of the epithelial cell into the peritubular capillary blood.

Some diuretics work by inhibiting the carbonic anhydrase enzyme. Inhibition of this enzyme prevents the formation of H ions within epithelial cells, which in turn reduces Na ion reabsorption. As indicated above (in the section Proximal Tubule Reabsorption of Salt and Water), if Na ion reabsorption is reduced, water reabsorption will also be reduced and a large volume of urine will result.

Loop of Henle Reabsorption of Salt and Water

- Descending limb of the loop of Henle is permeable to water but not to salt.
- Ascending limb of the loop of Henle is permeable to salt, because of a Na-K-Cl ion tritransporter, but not to water.
- Reabsorption of water from the descending limb results from the reabsorption of salt by the tritransporter in the ascending limb.

Tubular fluid leaving the proximal tubule is isotonic when it enters the descending limb of the loop of Henle but by the end of the loop, more salt than water is reabsorbed so that the fluid entering the distal tubule is hypotonic. This is the result of two things: the shape of the loop of Henle and the difference in permeability properties of the two limbs of the loop.

The epithelial cells of the ascending limb of the loop contain a tritransporter in the membrane on the luminal side of the cell. This tritransporter reabsorbs Na, K, and Cl ions together and is driven by the Na ion gradient as in the proximal tubule. The low water permeability of these epithelial cells and the action of the tritransporter enables the establishment of an osmotic gradient of 200 mOsm between the interstitial space and the tubular fluid of the ascending limb. The high osmolarity in the interstitial space generated by the tritransporter causes water to be reabsorbed from the fluid in the water-permeable descending limb of the loop.

Counter-current Multiplication

- An osmotic gradient is established in the interstitial space surrounding the loop of Henle that increases from the top to the bottom of the loop.
- The action of the tritransporter of the epithelial cells of the ascending limb, the water permeability of the descending limb, and the shape of the loop contribute to the development of this osmotic gradient.
- The process by which this occurs is called counter-current multiplication.

Counter-current multiplication derives its name from the fact that fluid moves in opposite directions in the two limbs of the loop of Henle and from the osmotic gradient in the interstitial space that increases from the top to the bottom of the loop. How counter-current multiplication results in this osmotic gradient is diagramed in a step-wise manner in Figure 4–6.

Assuming that initially all fluid within the loop has the same osmolarity (panel A) the tritransporter will reabsorb Na, K, and Cl from the tubular fluid creating an osmotic gradient of 200 mOsm between the interstitial space and the tubular fluid. The ascending limb is not permeable to water so water cannot follow. The descending limb is not permeable to salt so it cannot enter from the interstitial space. However, the descending limb is permeable to water so water is reabsorbed into the interstitial space. A new steady state is established (panel B). At this point new fluid enters from the proximal tubule displacing the fluid within the loop. This disrupts the steady state (panel C). Through the reabsorption of salt by the ascending limb and water by the descending limb, a new steady state is established (panel D). Notice that an osmotic gradient is being es-

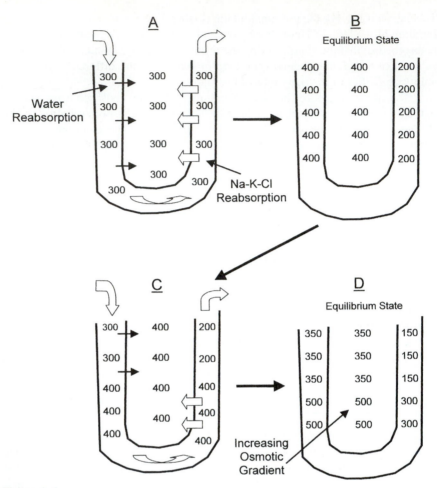

Figure 4–6
The shape and permeability properties of the loop of Henle enable an osmotic gradient to be established within the kidney. Diagrams A through D show in a step-wise manner how the gradient is established.

tablished in the interstitial space from the top to the bottom of the loop. It is the result of the loop structure and the different permeabilities of the two limbs of the loop. Fluid leaving the ascending limb is hypotonic compared to the fluid entering because more salt than water is reabsorbed. We will see in a later section that the interstitial osmotic gradient is critical for water reabsorption.

Distal Tubule Reabsorption of Salt and Water

- More salt than water is reabsorbed.
- Na and Cl ions reabsorbed together.

The distal tubule retains some of the properties of the ascending limb of the loop of Henle in that it is not very permeable to water and reabsorbs Na and Cl ions. The reabsorption of Na and Cl ions occurs through a co-transport carrier protein on the luminal side of the epithelial cell that combines the movement of one Na and one Cl ion into the cell. This reabsorption is driven by the Na ion concentration gradient established by the Na-K-ATPase on the basal lateral side of the epithelial cell.

Collecting Duct Reabsorption of Salt and Water

- The permeability of the collecting duct to Na ions and water is variable.
- Antidiuretic hormone (ADH) increases the permeability of the collecting duct to water.
- Aldosterone increases the reabsorption of Na ions by the collecting duct.

Na ions are reabsorbed by the epithelium of the collecting duct through protein channels in the luminal membrane. Na ions move through these channels into the epithelial cell because of a concentration gradient established by the Na-K-ATPase on the basal lateral membrane.

The collecting duct is sensitive to the effects of two hormones, *antidiuretic hormone (ADH)* and *aldosterone*. These two hormones regulate the ability of the collecting duct to reabsorb water and salt, respectively. In the absence of these two hormones, little salt and water is reabsorbed; but in their presence, reabsorption increases.

Antidiuretic hormone, also known as vasopressin, a posterior pituitary hormone, increases the number of *aquaporin channels* in the membrane of the epithelial cells increasing water reabsorption. Because the collecting duct passes from the cortex to the medulla of the kidney, it passes through the osmotic gradient established by the counter-current multiplication process of the loop of Henle. In the presence of ADH, water can leave the collecting duct in response to this osmotic gradient. In the absence of ADH it cannot.

Aldosterone, a hormone secreted by the adrenal cortex, acts on the collecting duct in several ways to increase Na reabsorption. Initially, it increases the number of Na ion channels that are open on the luminal membrane of the epithelial cells. If the level of aldosterone is sustained for several hours then the hormone induces the genetic expression of additional Na-K-ATPase molecules in the basal lateral side of the epithelial cells of the collecting duct. Both these effects enhance the reabsorption of Na ions.

Collecting Duct Secretion of K and H Ions

- The collecting duct secretes both K and H ions.
- K and H ion secretion is sensitive to aldosterone.

K ions are secreted through channels located in the luminal membrane of specialized epithelial cells of the collecting duct called *principle cells*. This secretion is down a concentration gradient established by the Na-K-ATPase located on the basolateral membrane. In the presence of aldosterone, more channels are opened and secretion is increased.

Specialized cells of the collecting duct, called *intercalated cells*, are responsible for H ion secretion. This secretion is due to an active transport process that moves H ions from the inside of the epithelial cell to the tubular fluid. The activity of this transporter is increased by aldosterone.

RENAL REGULATION OF SALT AND WATER BALANCE

Sensing Alterations in Salt Balance

- Salt balance, principally NaCl concentration, is assessed by monitoring osmolarity.
- Salt levels are changed by adjusting water reabsorption through the action of antidiuretic hormone.
- Antidiuretic hormone increases the number of open aquaporin channels in the collecting duct thereby increasing water reabsorption.

The body assesses the salt balance of the body by monitoring the osmolarity of the extracellular space. The primary osmotic agent in the extracellular space is the Na ion. Therefore, changes in osmolarity reflect changes in extracellular Na ion concentration.

Osmolarity is sensed by *osmoreceptors* in the hypothalamus. If NaCl concentration increases (extracellular osmolarity increases), water leaves the cells of the osmoreceptors in response to the increased extracellular osmolarity and they shrink. When these cells shrink, their electrical excitability increases and this stimulates the release of antidiuretic hormone (ADH) from the posterior pituitary. If the NaCl concentration decreases (extracellular osmolarity decreases), the cells of the osmoreceptors swell, their electrical activity decreases, and less ADH is released from the posterior pituitary.

ADH acts on the collecting duct. It increases water reabsorption of the collecting duct by increasing the number of open aquaporin channels in the epithelial cells. Because the collecting duct passes from the cortex to the medulla of the kidney through the osmotic gradient established by the loop of Henle, water is drawn from the permeable collecting duct as fluid flows along the tubule. In this way, the osmotic gradient generated by the counter-current multiplication system is exploited to increase water reabsorption. In the absence of ADH, the epithelial cells of the collecting duct are not permeable to water.

Sensing Alterations in Water Balance

- Water balance is assessed by monitoring blood volume through changes in blood pressure.
- Water levels are changed by adjusting salt reabsorption through the renin-angiotensin-II-aldosterone system.
- Increased sympathetic nerve stimulation directly increases renal secretion of renin.
- Decreased distal tubule Na-load directly stimulates renal renin secretion.
- Increased volume stimulates the secretion of atrial natriuretic peptide from the atria.

The body assesses its water balance by monitoring blood volume through both high- and low-pressure baroreceptors. The body interprets a fall in blood pressure as a fall in water volume and reflexes are initiated to restore this volume. The decreased stretch of the baroreceptors associated with a fall in blood pressure increases sympathetic nerve activity to the kidney. This stimulates the release of the enzyme *renin* from the kidney, which acts on a circulating peptide produced in the liver, *angiotensinogen,* to convert it to *angiotensin I.* Angiotensin-I is cleaved to *angiotensin-II* by an enzyme, *angiotensin converting enzyme (ACE),* located on the surface of endothelial cells. Angiotensin-II stimulates the adrenal cortex to release the hormone *aldosterone*, which stimulates Na^+ reabsorption by the collecting duct. Angiotensin-II also directly stimulates Na^+ reabsorption by cells of the proximal tubule. An increase in Na ion reabsorption adds Na^+ to the extracellular space, raising the extracellular osmolarity causing water to leave the cells of the body and expanding the extracellular volume.

Water balance is also monitored directly by the kidney through changes in Na ion delivery to the distal tubule. The fall in blood volume associated with water imbalance produces a fall in blood pressure, which limits GFR both directly and through the reflex mediated increase in sympathetic nerve stimulation. The lower GFR means that less Na ions are filtered and so fewer ions pass along the renal tubule to the distal tubule. When the Na ion concentration of the distal tubular fluid decreases, the distal tubular epithelial cells signal the cells of the afferent arterioles to release renin. This in turn leads to the formation of angiotensin-II and the secretion of aldosterone. This relationship between distal tubule Na^+ levels and renin secretion should not be confused with tubuloglomerular feedback discussed earlier. In this later feedback system, an increase in distal tubule Na^+ content stimulated the formation of an unknown vasoconstrictor that limited GFR.

If the fall in blood volume is sufficient (>10%), baroreceptor activation of the cardiovascular center (CV center) will be large enough to stimulate the release of ADH and renal water reabsorption will be increased.

If water volume increases, blood pressure rises and the baroreceptors are stimulated resulting in a decrease in sympathetic nerve activity and a decrease in the activity of the renin-angiotensin-II-aldosterone system. GFR increases both directly and through the reduced level of sympathetic nerve activity. This increases Na ion delivery to the distal tubule and reduces renin secretion. Also, the right atrium is stretched, which stimulates the release of the hormone, *atrial natriuretic peptide (ANP),* from atrial cells. ANP acts on the kidney to increase GFR and to inhibit renin release, both of which increase Na ion and, therefore, water excretion.

Reflex Response to Dehydration

- Dehydration initiates reflexes to conserve both salt and water.
- Dehydration reduces blood pressure, which reduces GFR and RBF independent of any other factors.
- Baroreceptor-initiated increased sympathetic nerve activity activates the renin-angiotensin-II-aldosterone system and decreases GFR and RBF.
- Osmoreceptors stimulate the release of ADH.
- Sense of thirst is stimulated.

Dehydration results from an imbalance between water intake and water loss. Such an imbalance can occur in the long distance runner training in the hot summer months. Sweat is hypotonic and so more water than salt is lost as the runner is cooled by evaporation. If insufficient water is consumed to replace the amount lost, dehydration occurs.

With sweating-induced dehydration, water volume decreases and osmolarity increases. The decrease in water volume causes the blood pressure to fall, which directly reduces GFR and RBF. This reduces both water and salt excretion by the kidney. The fall in blood pressure initiates a baroreceptor-mediated reflex response that includes increased sympathetic nerve activity to the kidney. Sympathetic nerve stimulation directly causes the release of renin from the kidney, which initiates the angiotensin-II-aldosterone system. In addition, sympathetic nerve stimulation produces afferent arteriolar constriction, which further reduces GFR and RBF and the excretion of Na^+ and water. Also, the fall in blood pressure directly reduces GFR and the distal tubule Na^+ load. The distal tubular epithelial cells stimulate the secretion of renin, which activates the angiotensin-II-aldosterone system. The elevated levels of aldosterone stimulate Na ion reabsorption, which further elevates the extracellular osmolarity and draws more water from the cells of the body to help increase extracellular volume.

The elevation in extracellular osmolarity resulting from the loss of water in sweat causes the cells of the osmoreceptors to shrink. This shrinkage stimulates the secretion of ADH from the posterior pituitary. ADH acting on the collecting duct epithelial cells increases water reabsorption.

These reflexes of the body are designed to reduce further fluid loss but do not replace the lost volume. However, with a loss of volume and an increase in osmolarity, a sense of thirst occurs. This occurs in part because angiotensin-II stimulates "thirst" centers in the brain initiating the sensation of thirst. In addition, higher centers also stimulate the sense of thirst independent of angiotensin-II. This increased drive for fluid intake helps replace the fluid that has been lost.

RENAL REGULATION OF ACID-BASE BALANCE
General Considerations

- Metabolism of food generates acid.
- Acid in the body is in two forms: fixed and volatile.
- Kidneys remove excess fixed acid; lungs remove excess volatile acid.
- Acidemia is excess H ions in the blood; alkalemia is excess bicarbonate ions in the blood.

The hydrogen ion concentration of body fluids is maintained between 3.8×10^{-8} and 4.17×10^{-8} M (pH = 7.38–7.42). However, each day 10 M of acid are produced in the form of CO_2 and 0.1 M are produced in the form of sulfuric and phosphoric acids. The body must excrete this large quantity of acid in order to keep the hydrogen ion concentration within normal limits.

Acid produced in the body is in two forms: volatile and fixed. Carbon dioxide is generated from the complete metabolism of food. Carbon dioxide combines with water to form hydrogen and bicarbonate ions according to the following chemical reaction:

$$CO_2 + H_2O \Leftrightarrow H_2CO_3 \Leftrightarrow H^+ + HCO_3^-.$$

This form of hydrogen ions is called *volatile acid* because blowing off or retaining CO_2 through the lungs can alter the amount of acid. Increasing ventilation will blow off more CO_2 driving the reaction to the left and lowering the H^+ concentration. Alternatively, decreasing ventilation will allow CO_2 to accumulate driving the reaction to the right and increasing the H^+ concentration. All other acid forms produced in the body are called *fixed acids*. These include sulfuric and phosphoric acids produced from sulfur containing amino acids and phospholipids, respectively.

The kidney has three roles in maintaining body hydrogen ion concentration. The first is to maintain an appropriate level of bicarbonate ions so that volatile acid can be formed. It does this by reabsorbing filtered bicarbonate and by synthesizing additional bicarbonate. Second, the kidney excretes the fixed acids produced by the body. Third, the kidney secretes hydrogen ions. The lungs help maintain the hydrogen ion concentration by adjusting the level of carbon dioxide through changes in ventilation as described earlier.

When the blood contains excess H ions the condition is called *acidemia,* and the process that produces the acidemia is called *acidosis.* When the blood contains excess bicarbonate ion, the condition is called *alkalemia,* and the process that produces the alkalemia is called *alkalosis.* Acidemia results either from the generation of excess H ions or the loss of bicarbonate, while alkalemia results from the generation of excess bicarbonate or the loss of H ions. A common cause of acidemia is diarrhea. Diarrhea fluid is alkaline and this loss of bicarbonate ions results in an excess of H ions in the blood (acidemia). Vomiting is a common cause of alkalemia. Vomitus is acidic and this loss of H ions results in excess bicarbonate ions in the blood (alkalemia).

Renal Production of Bicarbonate Ions

- The kidney produces bicarbonate through the formation of titratable acid.
- The kidney produces bicarbonate through the metabolism of glutamine.

Not only does the kidney reabsorb filtered bicarbonate, but it also generates additional bicarbonate. One way in which this occurs, is through the formation of *titratable acid* as illustrated in Figure 4–7. Fixed acids appear in the tubular fluid

TUBULAR FLUID

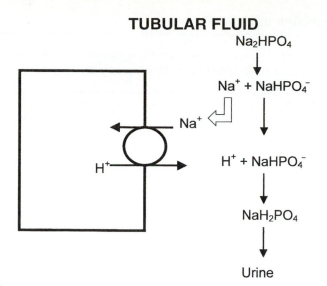

Figure 4–7

Formation of titratable acid in the proximal tubule is one way by which the kidney generates new bicarbonate ions in response to academia. The H^+ ion secreted by the epithelium is excreted as NaH_2PO_4 (titratable acid) leaving a bicarbonate ion behind.

because of filtration and are in the form of disodium salts. One of the Na ions can be reabsorbed in exchange for a secreted H ion, which converts the acid into a monosodium salt. As described earlier (see Figure 4–5), the H^+ for secretion is derived from the dissociation of carbonic acid. This means that the H ion that is excreted with the fixed acid leaves behind a bicarbonate ion. For every molecule of fixed acid excreted, a molecule of bicarbonate is added to the blood. To determine how much bicarbonate has been added, a urine sample is titrated with NaOH until the pH is 7.4. The NaOH converts the monosodium salt of the fixed acid back into the di-sodium form. The amount of NaOH needed to do this equals the amount of bicarbonate that was added to the blood. Because titration is used to make this determination, the fixed acid is called titratable acid.

The kidney also is able to generate bicarbonate ions through the metabolism of the amino acid, glutamine. Glutamine, produced in the liver, is converted to ammonium ions and α-ketoglutarate by the kidney. The ammonium ions are excreted, and the α-ketoglutarate is metabolized further by the kidney epithelial cells resulting in the production of bicarbonate ions. The bicarbonate ions pass across the basolateral membrane of the epithelial cell into the peritubular capillary blood.

Renal Secretion of H Ions

> • H ion secretion in the collecting duct leads to acidification of the urine.
> • Collecting duct H ion secretion is stimulated by aldosterone.

H ion secretion by the intercalated cells of the collecting duct, in contrast to cells of the proximal tubule, acidifies the urine. This is because collecting duct epithelial cells can generate a concentration gradient of H ions. The gradient exists because the epithelial cells are relatively impermeable to H ions and secrete H ions by means of an active transport pump located in the luminal membrane. Blood H ion concentration equals 4×10^{-8} M (pH = 7.4), but the collecting duct cells can increase the tubular fluid H ion concentration to 3×10^{-5} M (pH = 4.5), a concentration gradient of almost 1000 times.

The activity of the collecting duct H ion pump is influenced by aldosterone. Aldosterone stimulates the activity of the pump, increasing acid excretion.

Renal Compensation for Alkalemia

> Kidneys excrete bicarbonate and do not generate additional bicarbonate.

When the blood contains excess base, the kidney excretes bicarbonate and does not generate additional bicarbonate. Increased bicarbonate excretion occurs because there are insufficient H ions to be secreted by the proximal tubules to reabsorb all the filtered bicarbonate. The excess bicarbonate is excreted. Also, the low level of H ions means that filtered sulfuric and phosphoric acids will not be titrated and so no additional bicarbonate will be generated. In these ways, the kidney attempts to lower the blood bicarbonate concentration compensating for the alkalemia.

Renal Compensation for Acidemia

> Kidneys excrete H ions and generate additional bicarbonate.

When the blood contains excess H ions, the kidney excretes H ions and generates additional bicarbonate. In the presence of excess H ions, there are plenty of H ions to reabsorb all the filtered bicarbonate. In addition, the filtered fixed acids will be titrated generating additional bicarbonate ions. Also, the excess H ions stimulate the metabolism of glutamine by the kidney and the production of even more bicarbonate. Finally, the collecting duct increases its secretion of H ions. The combined effects of complete bicarbonate reabsorption, new bicarbonate generation, and the secretion of H ions helps the body compensate for the acidosis.

RENAL REGULATION OF K ION CONCENTRATION
Importance of a Constant Plasma K Ion Concentration

> Alterations in plasma K ion concentration produce cardiac arrhythmias.

Changes in the extracellular K ion concentration influence the membrane potential, which has the greatest impact on cardiac electrical activity. The resting membrane potential is determined by the transmembrane K ion concentration gradient. Raising the extracellular K ion concentration decreases the gradient producing depolarization and making the cell more excitable. Lowering the extracellular concentration does the opposite. These effects are most noticeable in the heart where small increases or decreases in extracellular K ion concentration lead to conduction problems potentially leading to cardiac arrest. The normal extracellular K ion concentration is 5 mM. A change of 2 mM is sufficient to result in cardiac conduction problems.

Renal Secretion of K Ions

> • Cortical collecting duct secretes K ions.
> • Secretion is stimulated by elevated plasma K ion or aldosterone concentrations.

The epithelial cells of the collecting duct secrete K ions. Secretion occurs through channels in the luminal membrane. The gradient for secretion is the result of the Na-K-ATPase on the basolateral membrane, which maintains a high intracellular K ion concentration. The ability to secrete potassium is a property of the *principal cells* of the collecting duct. These are distinct from the intercalated cells responsible for H ion secretion.

The plasma level of K^+ or aldosterone influences the amount of K^+ secreted by the principle cells. When plasma K^+ levels fall, secretion decreases and when it increases, so does secretion. This is because plasma K^+ concentration influences the activity of the Na-K-ATPase. An elevation in plasma K^+ levels stimulates the Na-K-ATPase causing more K^+ to enter the principal cell and providing more for secretion. The opposite occurs when plasma K ion levels decrease. Plasma K^+ levels are also sensed by the adrenal cortex. When plasma K^+ increases, aldosterone is secreted by the adrenal cortex. Aldosterone increases the number of open K^+ channels on the luminal membrane of the principal cell as well as the activity and number of Na-K-ATPase, which leads to increased K ion secretion.

Relationship Between Plasma K Ion Concentration and Acid-base Status

- Increases in plasma K^+ levels can lead to acidemia.
- Increases in plasma H ion concentration can lead to hyperkalemia.
- Plasma K^+ levels can compromise the ability of the kidney to regulate H ion excretion.

A relationship exists between the K and the H ion levels of the blood. When the plasma level of K^+ increases, movement of K^+ into cells is enhanced. To counter this movement of positive ions into the cell, H ions leave, raising the plasma H ion concentration and producing acidemia. So, *hyperkalemia* (elevated plasma K ion concentration) leads to acidemia. In an opposite manner, a fall in plasma K^+ concentration *(hypokalemia)* produces alkalemia.

Alternatively, changes in plasma H ion concentration influence plasma K^+ levels. An increase in H ion concentration (acidemia) causes K ions to leave cells, producing an increase in plasma K^+ levels or hyperkalemia. In an opposite manner, a fall in plasma H ion concentration (alkalemia) leads to hypokalemia.

Because of this relationship between plasma K and H ions, the plasma K^+ levels at the time of onset of either acidemia or alkalemia affect the ability of the kidney to compensate for the acid-base disturbance. For example, in the presence of a pre-existent hyperkalemia, the kidneys are less able to correct a subsequent acidosis from diarrhea because of the hyperkalemia-induced acidemia.

RENAL HANDLING OF CALCIUM AND PHOSPHATE

Renal Handling of Calcium

- All segments of the nephron reabsorb calcium except the descending limb of the loop of Henle.
- Reabsorption is influenced by parathyroid hormone and calcium levels.

All nephron segments except the descending limb of the loop of Henle reabsorb calcium (Ca). Calcium moves from the tubular fluid into the epithelial cells by passive diffusion down a concentration gradient. On the basal lateral side of the cells, it leaves either in exchange for Na ions or by means of an ATP-requiring calcium efflux pump.

The amount of calcium reabsorption is influenced by the plasma concentration of calcium and parathyroid hormone. An increase in plasma calcium levels reduces reabsorption, while an increase in parathyroid hormone leads to an increase in reabsorption.

Renal Handling of Phosphate

- Phosphate is reabsorbed in the proximal tubule coupled with sodium reabsorption.
- Phosphate reabsorption exhibits saturation.
- Parathyroid hormone inhibits renal phosphate reabsorption.

Phosphate reabsorption occurs in the proximal tubule. Reabsorption is coupled to the reabsorption of sodium ions (co-transport) as occurs with glucose and amino acids. The maximum capacity of this reabsorptive system is close to the amount of phosphate normally filtered. This means that an increase in plasma phosphate levels will increase the amount of filtered phosphate and exceed the capacity of the phosphate reabsorptive system. As a consequence, phosphate excretion is increased and normalization of plasma phosphate concentration occurs. Parathyroid hormone lowers the transport maximum of the Na–phosphate co-transporter, reducing phosphate reabsorption and increasing phosphate excretion.

RESPIRATORY PHYSIOLOGY

·

OVERVIEW OF LUNG FUNCTION AND STRUCTURE

Lung Functions

- Lungs are a site for gas exchange with the external environment.
- Regulate acid-base balance.
- Lungs are a defense mechanism.
- Lungs are a blood reservoir.
- Serve a biosynthetic function.

The lungs represent a site at which the external environment and the body intersect. The lung surface area is about the size of a tennis court, and so this point of intersection with the external environment is huge. This is both an advantage and a disadvantage. An advantage is that it is a point at which exchange can occur. The oxygen needed by the body can be obtained from inspired air, and carbon dioxide produced by the body can be released into expired air. Changes in ventilation match the oxygen supply with body demands. In addition, changes in ventilation can alter blood carbon dioxide levels and so alter the acid-base balance of the body.

However, a disadvantage of this interaction with the external environment is that the lungs are exposed to foreign substances. Therefore, the lungs are also a site of defense. The defense system exists at two levels. The first is to deal with inhaled particles. Depending upon their size, particles are either swept out of the airways entrapped in mucus or digested by macrophage. The second level of defense involves the immune system. Foreign organisms initiate an immunological response that includes invasion by white blood cells and the production of antibodies.

The lungs are a reservoir of blood that can be mobilized during times of reduced volume. Approximately 20% of the total blood volume resides in the pulmonary vasculature normally, but this volume can increase or decrease depending upon the output of the left ventricle.

Finally, the lungs also serve a biosynthetic function. They synthesize substances such as leukotrienes from arachidonic acid, convert substances to their active form like angiotensin-I to angiotensin-II, or degrade substances like norepinephrine and serotonin to an inactive form.

Lung Structure

- Lungs are composed of three basic elements: conducting airways, alveoli, and blood supply.
- Conducting airways enable air to reach alveoli and warm and humidify the air.
- Alveoli are blind sacs where gases in the inspired air exchange with the blood.
- Blood supply provides the heat and moisture to warm and humidify the inspired air and the nutrients for lung tissue, and it is the site of exchange between the body and inspired air.

Air is brought into the body through the *conducting airways*. This begins with the trachea, which divides into bronchi and subdivides multiple times into bronchioles. The conducting airways warm and humidify the inspired air but are not a site of gas exchange. The bronchioles end in sacs called *alveoli*. The alveoli are composed of a single layer of epithelial cells and are the site for gas exchange. The combined surface area of the alveoli is approximately that of a tennis court. The conducting airways and the alveoli are supplied with blood. The blood supply of the conducting airways provides the heat and moisture to warm and humidify the inspired air. It also provides for all the nutrient requirements of lung tissue. Finally, an elaborate capillary meshwork surrounds the alveoli enabling gas in the alveoli to exchange with gas in the blood.

MOVING AIR INTO AND OUT OF THE LUNGS (VENTILATION)

Lung–Chest Interaction

- Lungs are suspended within a closed chamber—the chest.
- Functional residual capacity is the equilibrium volume when the elastic forces of the chest wall and lungs are balanced.
- Changes in chest volume are responsible for changes in lung volume.

The lungs are suspended in a closed chamber—the chest. The chest consists of the rib cage and the diaphragm. The lungs are held against the chest wall by the surface tension of a thin layer of fluid, called the *pleural fluid*. Because of the natural elastic properties of the chest wall and lungs, the chest wall wants to expand and the lungs want to contract. The volume at which these two opposing forces balance is called the *functional residual capacity (FRC)*. At this volume the lungs and chest wall are in the "rest" position where forces are balanced and the pressure within the lungs equals atmospheric pressure. Inspiration begins from FRC.

These opposing forces generate a subatmospheric pressure within the space between the lungs and chest wall, the *intrapleural space*. This close apposition between the chest wall and the lungs makes the intrapleural space a closed space that is not connected to the outside air. Therefore, when the chest volume changes, the lungs are pulled along and their volume also changes.

Pressures in the Lungs and Chest

- Alveolar pressure is the pressure within the lungs.
- Intrapleural pressure is the pressure between the chest wall and the lungs.

The pressures within the lungs and chest are small in magnitude, being measured in centimeters of water rather than in millimeters of mercury. The pressure within the lungs is called the *alveolar pressure*. The pressure in the intrapleural space is called the *intrapleural pressure*.

Inspiration and Expiration

- Changes in chest volume are responsible for changes in lung volume.
- Diaphragm is the main muscle of inspiration.
- Contraction of the diaphragm increases chest volume inflating the lungs.

(continued)

> (*continued*)
> • Expiration is a passive process.
> • Muscles of the rib cage augment the action of the diaphragm.

The diaphragm is the main muscle of respiration under resting conditions. When relaxed, the diaphragm is dome-shaped. Upon contraction the dome flattens as the diaphragm descends causing the volume of the chest to increase (see Figure 5–1). Because the interior of the chest is closed to the atmosphere, this increase in volume causes the intrapleural pressure to fall and the lungs to be inflated. This expansion of the lungs lowers alveolar pressure so that it becomes less than atmospheric pressure and air is sucked into the lungs. At the end of an inspiration, alveolar pressure once again equals atmospheric pressure and airflow stops. When the diaphragm relaxes, it rises forming a dome, which lowers chest volume. This decrease in chest volume raises intrapleural pressure, causing alveolar pressure to increase above atmospheric, which pushes air out of the lungs. Therefore, expiration is a passive process.

When the volume of ventilation has to be increased, muscles of the chest wall help produce changes in chest volume beyond that produced by the contraction and relaxation of the diaphragm. Contraction of the external intercostal muscles helps increase the volume of the chest while contraction of the internal intercostal muscles helps to decrease chest volume.

Resistance to Air Flow

> • Medium-sized bronchi are the major site of resistance.
> • Autonomic nervous system and inspired irritants alter resistance.
> • Changes in lung volume alter resistance because bronchi are supported by lung tissue.

The medium-sized bronchi form the major site of resistance to air flow. The contractile activity of the bronchiolar smooth muscle is influenced by the autonomic nervous system. Sympathetic nerve stimulation causes relaxation and decreased resistance while parasympathetic nerve stimulation does the opposite. Irritants such as cigarette smoke cause an increase in resistance.

Because the bronchi are supported by surrounding lung tissue, changes in lung volume alter airway resistance. An increase in lung volume reduces resistance because the bronchi are pulled open. Patients with elevated airway resistance often breathe from an elevated FRC in an attempt to reduce the resistance.

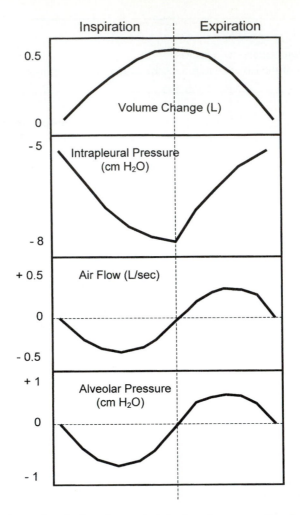

Figure 5–1
During inspiration and expiration, changes in intrapleural pressure alter alveolar pressure, which generates a pressure gradient leading to airflow and volume changes. The temporal relationship between these various parameters is illustrated in this figure.

Lung Volumes and Capacities

- Four terms describe specific volumes of the lungs: tidal, expiratory reserve, inspiratory reserve, residual
- Four terms describe lung capacities: functional residual, inspiratory, vital, total lung

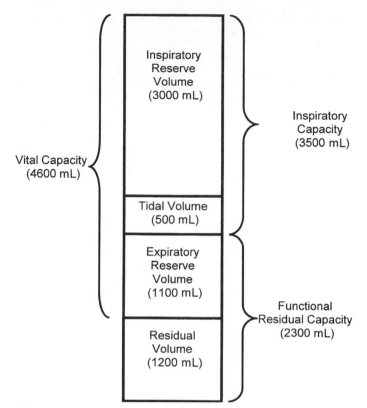

Figure 5–2
The quantity of air moved by the lung can be divided into various volumes and capacities. Their relationship to one another is diagramed in this figure.

The various volumes that the lung can assume are given specific names (see Figure 5–2). The change in lung volume needed to move air in and out is called *tidal volume (TV)*. During quiet breathing, tidal volume results from the contraction-relaxation of the diaphragm. The maximum lung volume that can be achieved above tidal volume is called *inspiratory reserve volume (IRV)*. The minimum lung volume that can be achieved below tidal volume is called *expiratory reserve volume (ERV)*. Like the heart, the lungs cannot be completely emptied. The amount of air remaining in the lungs after a forced expiration is called the *residual volume (RV)*.

The four lung volumes are combined in various ways to calculate four lung capacities.

$$\text{ERV} + \text{RV} = \textit{Functional residual capacity (FRC)}$$
$$\text{TV} + \text{IRV} = \textit{Inspiratory capacity (IC)}$$

$$ERV + TV + IRV = \textit{Vital capacity (VC)}$$
$$RV + ERV + TV + IRV = \textit{Total lung capacity (TLC)}$$

Dead Space Volumes

- Dead space is the volume of air that does not reach areas of the lung where gas exchange occurs.
- Anatomical dead space is due to the conducting airways.
- Alveolar dead space is due to alveoli that receive inadequate blood flow.
- Physiological dead space is the sum of anatomical and alveolar dead spaces.

Not all inspired air reaches areas of the lungs where gas exchange can occur. This volume of air is called *dead space volume*. Dead space volume has two components. One component, *anatomical dead space,* is due to basic lung anatomy in that the conducting airways are not designed for gas exchange. The volume of the conducting airways defines the volume of anatomical dead space. The second component of dead space volume is *alveolar dead space*. This volume represents the volume of gas that goes into alveoli that are not perfused with blood. The sum of anatomical and alveolar dead spaces is the *physiological dead space*.

Ventilation Is Uneven Within the Lungs

- The weight of the lungs produces uneven inflation of alveoli.
- Surfactant helps alveoli of different sizes remain inflated.

Not all alveoli are inflated to the same extent and this difference in inflation would be worse if it were not for the presence of surfactant.

The lungs are like a wet sponge hanging from the chest wall. When a person is in the upright position, the weight of the lungs pulls the lungs away from the chest wall at the top of the lungs and squeezes them against the chest wall at the base of the lungs. This means that intrapleural pressure is more negative at the top of the lungs and less negative at the base. As described in a previous section, alveolar volume depends on the difference between alveolar and intrapleural pressures. Alveolar pressure is the same everywhere in the lungs, but because of these regional differences in intrapleural pressure, alveoli at the top of the lungs are at a larger volume (more negative intrapleural pressure) than those at the base (less negative intrapleural pressure). So, at the beginning of a breath, some alveoli start at a larger volume than other alveoli.

As described for blood vessels, alveoli also exhibit a changing compliance as volume changes. At small volumes it takes a smaller pressure change to increase their volume (more compliant), while at larger volumes it takes a greater increase in pressure (less compliant). At the beginning of a breath, intrapleural pressure decreases the same amount everywhere. However, because the alveoli at the top of the lungs start at a larger volume, they are less compliant and consequently change their volume less with the same fall in intrapleural pressure. In contrast, alveoli at the base of the lung are more compliant because they start at a smaller volume. The same decrease in intrapleural pressure will cause their volume to increase more than those at the top of the lungs. Therefore, the weight of the lungs sets alveoli at different initial volumes, which affects how much their volume can be increased during a breath. Those at the base are ventilated more than those at the top of the lung.

The surface tension of alveoli would cause small alveoli to empty into larger alveoli if it were not for the effect of surfactant. The inner surface of the alveoli is coated with a thin layer of fluid. This fluid exerts a surface tension that tries to make the alveoli smaller. If this fluid was just water, the surface tension exerted in all alveoli would be the same regardless of their initial volume. Because the surface tension is trying to make the alveoli smaller, it is producing a pressure within the alveoli. The law of Laplace as written below, mathematically describes the relationship between pressure (P), radius (r), and surface tension (T).

$$P = T/r$$

As can be seen from this relationship, if surface tension is equal in all alveoli, those at small volumes (small r) will generate more pressure than those at large volumes. As a consequence, small alveoli will empty into large alveoli. This would generate large-volume alveoli, which from the previous discussion would be less compliant and more difficult to inflate. Fortunately, the fluid lining the alveoli contains *surfactant*, a phospholipid secreted by type II pneumocytes. Surfactant lowers the surface tension of alveoli and causes surface tension to change with volume. Small-volume alveoli have a small surface tension while large-volume alveoli have a large surface tension. This enables alveoli of unequal size to exist side-by-side.

Ventilation Equations

- Minute ventilation is the total volume of air moved into the lungs per unit time and equals the tidal volume times the breathing frequency ($MV = TV \times F$).
- Alveolar ventilation measures the volume of air that actually reaches the alveoli per unit time because it takes into account dead space volume [$V_A = (TV - DS) \times F$].
- Increasing tidal volume overcomes the effect of dead space volume.

The individual ventilation of each alveolus cannot be assessed but instead, the average ventilation of all alveoli is determined. Two relationships are used to express the magnitude of ventilation, *minute ventilation* and *alveolar ventilation*. Each measures a different aspect of ventilation.

The volume of air entering the lungs over time can be adjusted by varying the volume taken in with each breath or the number of breaths taken over time. The mathematical expression of this relationship is the *minute ventilation* and is given by the following equation:

$$\text{Minute ventilation } (MV) = \text{Tidal volume } (TV) \times \text{Breathing frequency } (F)$$

This relationship is analogous to the expression for cardiac output (CO = SV × HR) discussed in the cardiovascular chapter.

However, because of anatomical dead space, not all inspired air reaches the alveoli. To determine this volume, minute ventilation has to be corrected for dead space volume. When this is done, *alveolar ventilation* is obtained, which is given by the following equation:

$$\text{Alveolar ventilation } (\dot{V}_A) = (\text{Tidal volume} - \text{Dead space volume}) \times F$$
$$= (TV - DS) \times F$$

Examination of these two equations indicates that various combinations of tidal volume and breathing frequency can produce the same minute ventilation but not the same alveolar ventilation. The following table illustrates this point assuming a dead space of 150 mL.

TIDAL VOLUME (mL)	F (breaths/min)	MV (mL/min)	$\dot{V}_A$ (mL/min)
300	20	6000	3000
500	12	6000	4200
600	10	6000	4500
150	40	6000	0

The greater the tidal volume, the less of the total volume will be taken up by the dead space volume. At the extreme, no matter how fast one breathes, if tidal volume does not exceed the dead space volume, alveolar ventilation will be zero and no gas exchange will be possible. Animals make use of this situation when they pant. Shallow rapid breaths are taken, which enables heat radiated by the conducting airways to be removed while not altering the gas composition of the blood because no alveolar ventilation occurs.

MOVEMENT OF GAS BETWEEN ALVEOLAR AIR AND BLOOD

General Considerations

- Driving force for gas movement is the difference in gas partial pressure.
- Diffusion and blood flow influence the amount of a gas in the blood.

Gas movement between alveolar air and blood is a passive process determined by the concentration gradient for the particular gas. In a gas mixture such as air, each gas exerts a pressure that is related to the proportion of gas in the mixture. At sea level the gases in the air exert a total pressure of 760 mm Hg. Oxygen represents 21% of the air and, therefore, exerts a pressure of 160 mm Hg (21% of 760 mm Hg). This pressure is called the *partial pressure* and for oxygen would be abbreviated, Po_2. The sum of the partial pressures of each gas in the air at sea level equals 760 mm Hg.

A gas will move from an area where its partial pressure is high to one where it is low. At the interface between a gas and a liquid, a gas will move between these two media until its partial pressure is equal in the gas and the liquid. In the lung, gases move between alveolar air and the blood based on their partial pressure. Gas will move from alveolar air to blood if its partial pressure in alveolar air is greater than in the blood. If the partial pressure of the gas is greater in blood then in alveolar air, it will move into alveolar air. Normally, the partial pressure of oxygen is high and the partial pressure of carbon dioxide is low in alveolar air. The opposite is true for the partial pressures of these gases in the blood entering the lungs. It is these differences in partial pressures that produce the driving force for oxygen to enter the blood and carbon dioxide to leave the blood as blood flows through the alveolar capillary bed.

The gas partial pressure provides the driving force but two things determine the effectiveness of this driving force. The first is how fast a particular gas can diffuse between the two compartments. Gases do not all diffuse at the same rate, which is determined by various physical factors (see Physical Factors Affect Gas Diffusion). The second determinant of the amount of gas moving is the rate of blood flow (see Blood Flow Affects the Amount of Gas in the Blood). When diffusion is not limiting, the rate of blood flow determines how much of a gas is delivered to or carried from the alveoli and, therefore, the amount of gas that can move into or out of the blood.

Gas Composition of Alveolar Air

- Partial pressures of oxygen and carbon dioxide in alveolar air are not the same as those in atmospheric air.
- Humidification lowers the P_{O_2} of inspired air.
- P_{O_2} of alveolar air is lower than inspired air because of uptake by the blood.
- Carbon dioxide diffusing from pulmonary arterial blood into alveolar air raises alveolar P_{CO_2} compared to that of inspired air.

At sea level (760 mm Hg), air is composed primarily of nitrogen and oxygen and little if any carbon dioxide. As described above, oxygen represents 21% of the gases in air so it exerts a partial pressure of 160 mm Hg. Since there is essentially no carbon dioxide in air, it exerts no partial pressure. As air is drawn into the lungs and passes down the conducting airways, it is humidified. The water vapor becomes part of the total gas in inspired air and exerts a partial pressure of 47 mm Hg at body temperature. This reduces the P_{O_2} to 150 mm Hg because now oxygen occupies 21% of a lower available gas pressure $[21\% \times (760-47)]$. When inspired air reaches the alveoli, the P_{O_2} is reduced further to approximately 100 mm Hg because of the uptake of oxygen by the blood.

The P_{O_2} of alveolar air at any moment is determined by the rate of ventilation and removal by the pulmonary blood. When the oxygen consumption of the body increases, both ventilation and pulmonary blood flow increase to meet the body's needs. We will see in a later section (Balancing Ventilation and Perfusion) that the balance between ventilation and blood flow within the normal lung is not perfectly matched. This imbalance will generate regional differences in P_{O_2}.

The P_{CO_2} of inspired air is zero but that of alveolar air is 40 mm Hg. This is because carbon dioxide produced by the body and carried to the alveoli by pulmonary arterial blood diffuses into the alveolar air raising its P_{CO_2}. The balance between ventilation and blood flow also determines alveolar P_{CO_2}. During periods of increased activity, tissues of the body produce more carbon dioxide and in response, the body increases ventilation and pulmonary blood flow to remove this excess carbon dioxide.

Physical Factors Affect Gas Diffusion

- Fick's law of diffusion relates four factors that determine the amount of gas transferred through a sheet of tissue: cross-sectional area, partial pressure, diffusion constant, and thickness.
- Diffusion constant is related to the gas solubility and molecular weight.
- Movement of oxygen and carbon dioxide are not limited by diffusion.

Four factors determine the amount of gas diffusing through a sheet of tissue over time, but only one changes under normal conditions. The four factors are the surface area of the tissue, the difference in the partial pressure of the gas on either side of the tissue surface, the thickness of the tissue, and the diffusion constant. The amount of gas diffusing will increase if the surface area or the difference in partial pressures increases. However, if the tissue thickness increases, then the amount of gas diffusing decreases. The diffusion constant relates two physical properties of the gas, which are the solubility of the gas and its molecular weight. The greater the solubility and the smaller the molecular weight, the larger is the diffusion constant and, therefore, the more gas will diffuse through.

Of these, only the gas partial pressure changes under normal conditions. Surface area and tissue thickness only change with disease. During exercise for example, the partial pressure of oxygen decreases and the partial pressure of carbon dioxide increases in venous blood. These changes enhance the diffusion of oxygen from alveolar air into the blood and carbon dioxide from the blood into alveolar air.

Fick's law is a mathematical expression of these factors.

Gas diffusion is proportional to

$$\frac{\text{Surface area} \times \text{Diffusion constant} \times \text{Partial pressure gradient}}{\text{Thickness}}$$

The physical properties of oxygen and carbon dioxide enable them to diffuse rapidly between the alveolar air and the blood. Therefore, the amount of these gases in the blood is not limited by diffusion. As described in the next section, blood flow limits that amount of these gases in the blood.

Blood Flow Affects the Amount of Gas in the Blood

> • The amount of gas dissolved in blood can be limited by pulmonary blood flow.
> • The amount of oxygen and carbon dioxide in the blood is limited by perfusion.

In addition to diffusion, blood flow can limit the amount of a gas that is in the blood. It takes about three quarters of a second for blood to flow through a pulmonary capillary. Within one quarter of a second, oxygen in the alveolar air equilibrates with that in the blood. This means that during the remaining half of a second that the blood is in the alveolar capillary, it will not take on more oxygen. This means that the amount of oxygen being carried by the blood to the rest of the body will depend upon how fast the blood flows through the pulmonary capillaries. Since each volume of blood has equilibrated with alveolar oxygen, the more volumes that pass through the pulmonary capillaries the more oxygen will be delivered to the rest of the body. For this reason, oxygen is said to be *perfusion limited*. The removal of carbon dioxide from the blood is also perfusion limited. Only when blood flow becomes so rapid that it takes less than a one quarter second to pass through a pulmonary capillary will diffusion of oxygen or carbon dioxide affect the amount of these gasses in the blood.

MOVEMENT OF BLOOD THROUGH THE LUNGS

Overview of Pulmonary Blood Flow and Resistance

> • The volume of blood flow through the lungs is the same as through the systemic circulation but because the resistance is lower, pressure is lower too.
> • Pulmonary vascular resistance is increased by norepinephrine, serotonin, and histamine; adenosine, acetylcholine, and nitric oxide decrease resistance.
> • Reduced alveolar oxygen causes increased pulmonary vascular resistance.

The outputs of the right and left ventricles are equal when averaged over several heartbeats. Therefore, the volume of blood flow through the pulmonary and systemic circulations is identical. However, the pulmonary vascular resistance is about one tenth the resistance of the systemic circulation, so the same blood flow can be produced by a smaller pressure gradient. The pressure difference between the right ventricle and the left atrium is only about 10 mm Hg.

The pulmonary vasculature is poorly innervated and so circulating chemical agents primarily influence its resistance. Norepinephrine, serotonin, and histamine all increase resistance while adenosine, acetylcholine, and nitric oxide decrease resistance. Interestingly, reduced alveolar oxygen *(hypoxia)* causes increased resistance. This is opposite to its effect on systemic vessels. The mechanism by which reduced oxygen causes vasoconstriction is not known. However, it makes sense because one would want to reduce the blood flow to alveoli with low oxygen so that the blood could be directed toward those with more oxygen.

Lung Volume Affects Pulmonary Vascular Resistance

> Pulmonary vascular resistance increases at both small and large lung volumes because alveolar and extra-alveolar vessels are affected differently by changes in lung volume.

The resistance of alveolar and extra-alveolar vessels is affected differently by changes in lung volume. *Alveolar vessels* are the capillaries associated with each alveolus. *Extra-alveolar vessels* are all the other vessels supplying lung tissue. Because the capillaries are not supported by connective tissue, their caliber is influenced by alveolar volume. At large lung volumes (ie, large alveolar volume) capillaries are compressed, which raises their resistance to blood flow. On the other had, extra-alveolar vessels have thick walls whose natural elasticity tends to reduce their diameter. They are held at a larger diameter by lung connective tissue. At large lung volumes, the connective tissue is stretched, opposing the tendency of the extra-alveolar vessels to narrow. However, at small lung volumes the connective tissue is not stretched, allowing the extra-alveolar vessels to narrow. Therefore, resistance is high at low lung volumes because of extra-alveolar vessel narrowing, while at large lung volume resistance increases because of alveolar vessel narrowing.

Blood Flow Is Uneven Within the Lungs

> Gravity causes blood pressure and therefore blood flow to be greater at the base than at the top of the lung.

Just as gravity produces regional differences in alveolar inflation (see Ventilation Is Uneven in the Lungs), it also produces regional differences in blood flow. In a person standing upright, the weight of the column of blood from the top to the bottom of the lung is about 20 mm Hg. This additional pressure at the base of the lungs enhances blood flow in this region. Therefore, the effect of gravity is to produce regional differences in blood flow that increase from the top to the bottom of the lung.

BALANCING VENTILATION AND PERFUSION
Normal Ventilation–Perfusion Imbalance

> - Regional differences in ventilation and blood flow cause the top of the lung to be overventilated and the bottom of the lung to be overperfused under normal conditions.
> - Regional differences in the ratio of ventilation to perfusion result in regional differences in gas exchange from the top to the bottom of the normal lung.
> - Because of ventilation–perfusion imbalance, blood leaving the top of the lung has a higher P_{O_2} and a lower P_{CO_2} than blood leaving the base of the lung.

On the average, the ratio of alveolar ventilation ($\dot{V}_A$) to cardiac output (CO or $\dot{Q}$), the *ventilation-perfusion ratio ($\dot{V}_A/\dot{Q}$)*, is approximately one. However, as described in previous sections, the effect of gravity produces differences in ventilation and perfusion from the top to the bottom of the lung (see Figure 5–3). Relative to the top of the lung, the base of the lung is ventilated (approximately 3×) and perfused (approximately 19×) better. However, because the change in ventilation from the top to the bottom of the lung is not as great as the change in blood flow, $\dot{V}_A/\dot{Q}$ decreases from the top to the bottom of the lung (approximately 5×). This means that the top of the lung is overventilated relative to its blood flow, and the base of the lung is overperfused relative to its ventilation. In other words, $\dot{V}_A/\dot{Q}$ is high at the top of the lung and low at the base of the lung. This imbalance between alveolar ventilation and blood flow is also called $\dot{V}$-$\dot{Q}$ *mismatch*.

Because of regional differences in $\dot{V}_A/\dot{Q}$, gas exchange also varies from the top to the bottom of the lung. The consequence of a high $\dot{V}_A/\dot{Q}$ is to increase the partial pressure of oxygen and decrease the partial pressure of carbon dioxide of the alveolar capillary blood. The opposite occurs with a low ventilation-perfusion ratio. Therefore, blood leaving the alveoli in the top of the lung has a higher oxygen partial pressure and a lower carbon dioxide partial pressure than blood leaving the base of the lung. When blood from all regions of the lung combines to form the mixed venous blood leaving the lungs, the oxygen partial pressure of the blood is less than that in mixed alveolar air. This difference is called the *alveolar–arterial oxygen difference*. Normally this difference is very small (approximately 4 mm Hg), but it increases with lung disease.

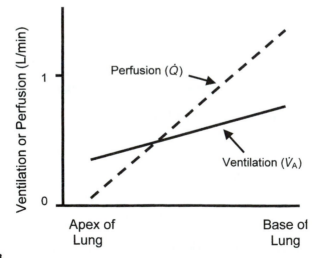

Figure 5–3
Because of the effect of gravity, lung perfusion ($\dot{Q}$), and ventilation ($\dot{V}_A$) increase from the top (apex) to the bottom (base) of the lung.

Shunts

- "Shunt" is a term used to describe a condition in which V_A/Q is zero due to no ventilation.
- Anatomical shunts result from blood vessels that do not flow past alveoli.
- Alveolar shunts result from alveoli that are not ventilated or are not capable of exchanging gas.
- A physiological shunt is the sum of anatomical and alveolar shunts.
- The greater the magnitude of the physiological shunt, the lower the P_{O_2} and the higher the P_{CO_2} of arterial blood.
- The greater the magnitude of the physiological shunt, the greater the alveolar–arterial oxygen difference.

Shunt refers to a condition in which V_A/Q is zero because of no ventilation. The lack of ventilation occurs for two reasons: Either the vasculature does not have access to alveoli or alveoli do not permit gas exchange because they are either physically plugged (not ventilated) or impermeable to gas.

Shunts exist normally. For example, some of the arterial blood perfusing the bronchi goes directly into pulmonary veins without passing through the lungs. This type of shunt, caused by the structural organization of the vasculature, is called an *anatomical shunt.* On the other hand, if the alveoli are unable to exchange gas due to blockage or impermeability, the shunt is called an *alveolar shunt.* The combined effect of anatomical and alveolar shunts is called a *physiological shunt.*

The net effect of a physiological shunt is to essentially mix venous blood (blood that has not had a chance to undergo alveolar gas exchange) with arterial blood (blood that has undergone alveolar gas exchange). The consequence of this mixing is that the P_{O_2} of arterial blood decreases and the P_{CO_2} increases, which also increases the alveolar–arterial oxygen difference.

Shunts and Dead Space Are Related and Represent the Limits of $\dot{V}_A/\dot{Q}$

- Shunts refer to conditions where $\dot{V}_A/\dot{Q}$ is zero because of no ventilation, whereas dead space refers to conditions where $\dot{V}_A/\dot{Q}$ is infinite because of no blood flow.
- Both shunts and dead space have anatomical and alveolar components.
- Shunts and dead space represent the limits of $\dot{V}_A/\dot{Q}$.

Shunts and dead space are related and describe specific extremes of the $\dot{V}_A/\dot{Q}$ ratio. As we have just seen, *shunt* refers to a $\dot{V}_A/\dot{Q}$ that is zero due to no ventilation. In contrast, *dead space* refers to a $\dot{V}_A/\dot{Q}$ that is infinite because blood flow is zero. Remember that dead space represents those areas of the lung that are ventilated but not perfused (see Dead Space Volumes above). In these areas $\dot{V}_A/\dot{Q}$ is infinite. Also, both shunts and dead space are comprised of anatomical and alveolar components that when combined are called either physiological shunts or physiological dead space.

On a continuum of $\dot{V}_A/\dot{Q}$ ratios, shunts and dead space represent the limits. One can imagine the ratio moving through a series of values from one extreme where ventilation is zero to another where blood flow is zero. If one plots alveolar P_{CO_2} as a function of alveolar P_{O_2}, the impact on gas exchange of $\dot{V}_A/\dot{Q}$ ratios between shunt and dead space can be seen (see Figure 5–4). In the presence of a shunt, alveolar air has the gas composition of venous blood ($P_{CO_2} = 46$ mm Hg; $P_{O_2} = 40$ mm Hg) because it has not been altered by exchange with outside air. At the other extreme, dead space, alveolar air has the gas composition of inspired air ($P_{O_2} = 150$ mm Hg; $P_{CO_2} = 0$) because it has not been altered by exchange with venous blood. Between these extremes where there is some degree of ventilation and perfusion, alveolar air and, therefore, pulmonary blood will have a P_{CO_2} and a P_{O_2} between these limits.

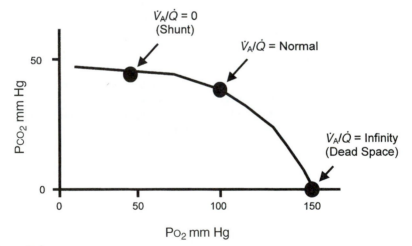

Figure 5–4
Mismatches in the ventilation to perfusion ratio ($\dot{V}_A/\dot{Q}$) affect the partial pressures of oxygen and carbon dioxide in alveolar air. In ventilated alveoli, as the level of perfusion decreases to zero (dead space), the oxygen partial pressure increases and the carbon dioxide partial pressure decreases. In perfused alveoli, as ventilation decreases to zero (shunt), the oxygen partial pressure decreases and the carbon dioxide partial pressure increases.

OXYGEN AND CARBON DIOXIDE TRANSPORT BY THE BLOOD

Gas Composition of Arterial and Venous Blood

- Systemic arterial and pulmonary venous blood are high in oxygen and low in carbon dioxide.
- Systemic venous and pulmonary arterial blood are high in carbon dioxide and low in oxygen.

Because in alveolar air the P_{O_2} is high and the P_{CO_2} is low, blood leaving the lungs (pulmonary venous blood) is high in oxygen and low in carbon dioxide relative to the blood entering the lungs (pulmonary arterial blood). Pulmonary venous blood flows into the left atrium and is then pumped out the left ventricle as systemic arterial blood. When the systemic arterial blood reaches capillary beds in the various tissues of the body, oxygen leaves and carbon dioxide is acquired. This lowers the P_{O_2} and increases the P_{CO_2} of systemic venous blood returning to the right atrium. The right ventricle pumps this blood (pulmonary arterial blood) through the lungs. In the lungs the partial pressures of oxygen and carbon dioxide in blood and alveolar air favors the movement of carbon dioxide into alveolar air and oxygen into blood. The direction of these exchanges and gas partial pressures are illustrated in Figure 5–5.

Oxygen Transport in the Blood

- Oxygen is carried in two forms: dissolved and bound to hemoglobin.
- Dissolved oxygen is inadequate to meet the body's needs.
- Hemoglobin greatly increases the blood's oxygen-carrying capacity.
- Three terms describe the amount of oxygen in the blood: capacity, saturation, content.
- Oxygen binding to hemoglobin is influenced by pH, carbon dioxide, 2,3-diphosphoglycerate, and temperature.
- Carbon monoxide decreases the blood's oxygen content and capacity.

Oxygen is carried in two forms in the blood: dissolved and bound to hemoglobin. The amount that can be dissolved in arterial blood is directly related to the P_{O_2} to which it is exposed in the lungs. At normal alveolar P_{O_2} (100 mm Hg), there is 0.3 mL of dissolved O_2/100 mL of blood (see Figure 5–6). When the blood reaches the tissue, oxygen consumption reduces the dissolved oxygen to 0.12 mL/100 mL of blood ($P_{O_2} = 40$ mm Hg). This means that 0.18 mL of oxygen/100 mL of blood

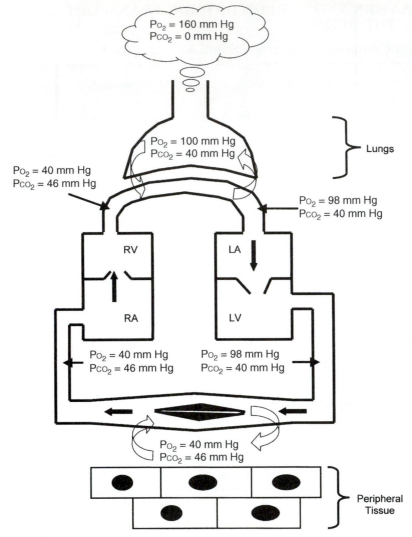

Figure 5–5
Movement of carbon dioxide and oxygen between the alveolar air and the blood and between the blood and peripheral tissue depends upon the concentration gradients for these gases. As can be seen in this figure, the gradients favor the movement of oxygen from alveolar air to the tissue and the movement of carbon dioxide from the tissue to alveolar air.

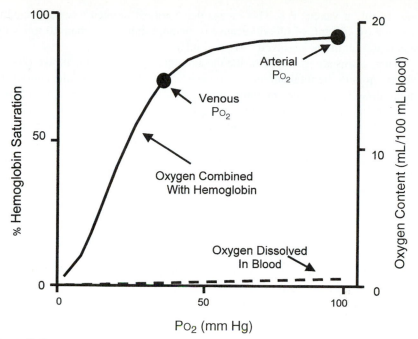

Figure 5–6
Oxygen is present in the blood in a dissolved form and is bound to hemoglobin. The partial pressure of oxygen determines how much is in each form. Much more oxygen is bound to hemoglobin at any partial pressure than is dissolved.

have been released. At a resting blood flow of 5 L/min, 9 mL of oxygen/min are delivered to the tissue in dissolved form. However, resting oxygen consumption is 250 mL/min so the body must have a more effective way to deliver oxygen to metabolizing tissue.

Hemoglobin enables the blood to carry large quantities of oxygen. Hemoglobin consists of a heme, an iron-prophyrin, bound to a globin molecule, a large polypeptide chain. Four heme-globin complexes combine to form the whole hemoglobin molecule. There are 4 different globin molecules that vary slightly in amino acid composition and are designated alpha, beta, gamma, and delta chains. The most common form is hemoglobin A, which consists of 2 alpha and 2 beta chains. Oxygen binds to the iron atoms in hemoglobin and because the molecule contains 4 iron atoms, 4 oxygen molecules can be bound.

The amount of bound oxygen depends on the P_{O_2} and is described by the oxygen-hemoglobin binding curve shown in Figure 5–6. Notice that at normal arterial P_{O_2} (100 mm Hg), hemoglobin is over 95% saturated and that even at normal venous P_{O_2} (40 mm Hg) it is still 75% saturated. Because of hemoglobin, 100 mL of blood contain approximately 19 mL of oxygen at arterial P_{O_2} and about 14 mL at venous P_{O_2}. This means that 5 mL of oxygen were delivered to the tissue by 100 mL of blood because of hemoglobin, more than 10 times the amount present in the dissolved form (0.3 mL).

Three terms are used to describe the amount of oxygen in the blood. *Oxygen content* refers to the total amount of oxygen in the blood, that is, the sum of the amount dissolved plus the amount bound to hemoglobin. Two terms describe the amount of oxygen combined with hemoglobin. The first of these is *oxygen capacity*, which is the maximum amount of oxygen that can combine with hemoglobin. It is determined by exposing blood to a very high P_{O_2} and calculating the amount bound to hemoglobin after subtracting the amount dissolved. The oxygen capacity is determined by the amount of hemoglobin in the blood and by the ability of hemoglobin to bind oxygen. The final term used to describe the amount of oxygen bound to hemoglobin is *oxygen saturation*. Oxygen saturation is the proportion of the total number of oxygen binding sites that are occupied. It is determined by the P_{O_2} and the ability of hemoglobin to bind oxygen, but not by the amount of hemoglobin present in the blood.

The oxygen content of blood and the oxygen capacity and saturation of hemoglobin are influenced by physiological and pathological factors. As arterial blood circulates past metabolically active tissue, the hydrogen ion concentration, P_{CO_2}, and temperature of the blood increase. These changes reduce the ability of hemoglobin to bind oxygen (decreasing oxygen saturation and content) at any P_{O_2} and enhance the amount of oxygen released for tissue consumption. When the blood reaches the lungs, hydrogen ion concentration and the P_{CO_2} decrease enhancing the binding of oxygen to hemoglobin. Red blood cells produce 2,3-diphosphoglycerate (2,3-DPG) because they cannot metabolize aerobically since they lack mitochondria. 2,3-DPG binds to hemoglobin and decreases oxygen binding. During chronically low P_{O_2}, 2,3-DPG increases enabling hemoglobin to release more oxygen.

Inhalation of carbon monoxide (CO) has several effects on oxygen transport by the blood. The affinity of CO for hemoglobin is 240 times that for oxygen, so very small amounts of CO will occupy a large number of the oxygen binding sites. This effectively reduces the oxygen capacity of hemoglobin. Because of this, hemoglobin becomes saturated with oxygen at very low P_{O_2} values, values that are less than those in venous blood. This means that little if any oxygen will be released for tissue use. The net effect is that at normal alveolar P_{O_2} oxygen content and capacity of blood is greatly reduced even though hemoglobin is saturated and the amount of dissolved oxygen is normal.

Carbon Dioxide Transport by Blood

• Carbon dioxide is transported in the blood in three forms: dissolved, as bicarbonate, and bound to hemoglobin.

(continued)

(*continued*)
• Blood contains more carbon dioxide than it does oxygen.
• Carbon dioxide binding to hemoglobin is affected by P_{O_2}.

Carbon dioxide is carried in the blood as dissolved gas, in the form of bicarbonate ions, and bound to hemoglobin. Of the three, most carbon dioxide is carried in the form of bicarbonate ions. Carbon dioxide diffuses into red blood cells where it combines with water to form carbonic acid under the influence of the enzyme *carbonic anhydrase*. Carbonic acid spontaneously dissociates into hydrogen and bicarbonate ions. The hydrogen ions bind to hemoglobin and the bicarbonate ions diffuse from the red blood cells into the plasma. Depending upon the P_{CO_2}, 60 to 90% of the carbon dioxide is converted to bicarbonate ions by this mechanism. In addition, some (5–30% depending upon P_{CO_2}) of the carbon dioxide inside red blood cells binds to the globin portion of the hemoglobin molecule to form carbamino compounds.

Over the normal P_{CO_2} range (40–45 mm Hg), the blood carbon dioxide content is greater than that for oxygen (see Figure 5–7).

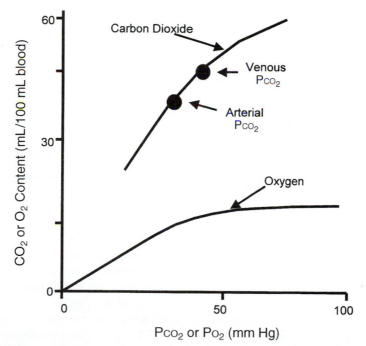

Figure 5–7
The blood carries much more carbon dioxide than oxygen.

Just as carbon dioxide alters oxygen binding to hemoglobin, oxygen alters carbon dioxide binding. As the P_{O_2} increases, less carbon dioxide can bind to hemoglobin. This interrelationship between oxygen and carbon dioxide binding to hemoglobin facilitates gas exchange with hemoglobin both in the lungs and in the tissue. In the lungs, P_{O_2} is high, which reduces carbon dioxide binding to hemoglobin, facilitating release into alveolar air. In the tissue P_{O_2} is low, which increases carbon dioxide binding to hemoglobin, facilitating its removal from the tissue. As described in the previous section (Oxygen Transport in the Blood) changes in P_{CO_2} facilitate oxygen binding to hemoglobin in an appropriate manner in tissue and lung.

CONTROL OF VENTILATION

Control of Breathing Rhythm

- Medulla and pons form the integration center and contain neural elements that define the basic breathing rhythm.
- Afferent input from higher brain centers and lung receptors modulate the basic rhythm.
- Primary efferent output is via the phrenic nerve to the diaphragm.

The medulla and pons contain neural elements that are sufficient to maintain rhythmic breathing. Transecting the brain above the pons does not modify the basic breathing rhythm, while transecting below the medulla stops the rhythm. Within these areas are groups of neurons called the *ventral respiratory group* and the *dorsal respiratory group* that are responsible for establishing this rhythm.

The basic rhythm is modulated by higher brain centers and by receptors located in the chest wall and lungs. Higher brain centers alter the basic respiratory rhythm in a variety of circumstances such as when you are talking or experiencing fear and anger. In the lungs and chest wall there are receptors that sense stretch and the presence of irritants. Stretch receptors provide information about the volume of the lungs. If information from these receptors is blocked, the depth of respiration increases. Irritant receptors are involved in initiating a cough and for sensing pain. The vagus nerve carries all afferent signals from these receptors to the brain.

The phrenic nerve is responsible for stimulating contraction of the diaphragm. Neural signals from the medulla stimulate the phrenic nerve, which exits the spinal cord at the third to fifth cervical level and travels to the skeletal muscles of the diaphragm. Changing the activity of the phrenic nerve changes the depth and frequency of respiration. Motor nerves that exit the spinal cord at several levels in the thorax innervate intercostal muscles. These muscles are activated when large volumes of air must be moved.

Ventilation Influenced by P_{O_2}, P_{CO_2}, and pH

- Two groups of chemoreceptors, medullary and peripheral, send afferent information to the medulla and influence the depth and rate of respiration.
- Medullary chemoreceptors are sensitive to pH and increase ventilation when pH falls.
- Peripheral chemoreceptors are sensitive to pH, P_{O_2}, and P_{CO_2} with P_{CO_2} being most effective.
- Sensitivity of the peripheral chemoreceptors is influenced by pH, P_{O_2}, and P_{CO_2}.

Chemoreceptors are located in the medulla of the brain and in the periphery on the carotid arteries and aortic arch. Each receptor is sensitive to different substances in the blood. The *medullary chemoreceptors* or *central chemoreceptors* are sensitive to pH while the *peripheral chemoreceptors* are sensitive to the pH, P_{O_2}, and P_{CO_2} of arterial blood.

Since the blood-brain barrier is impermeable to H^+, the medullary chemoreceptors do not directly sense the pH of the blood. However, CO_2 can diffuse from the blood into the cerebral spinal fluid where it is converted to H^+ and HCO_3^-. The hydrogen ions thus formed stimulate the medullary chemoreceptors. Therefore, these receptors really monitor the P_{CO_2} of arterial blood by sensing changes in the pH of the cerebral spinal fluid. A decrease in pH (an increase in P_{CO_2}) will stimulate the receptor and increase ventilation. The increased ventilation will blow off the CO_2 lowering the arterial P_{CO_2} and the cerebral spinal fluid hydrogen ion concentration. Because of the need for the chemical conversion of CO_2 to H^+, the receptors are slow to respond to changes in arterial pH.

The peripheral chemoreceptors are located on both carotid arteries and the aorta in special structures called *carotid and aortic bodies*. The peripheral chemoreceptors directly respond to changes in arterial pH, P_{O_2}, and P_{CO_2}. The carotid body chemoreceptors are sensitive to all three while the aortic body is not sensitive to P_{O_2}. The receptors are active at normal levels of arterial pH, P_{O_2}, and P_{CO_2}. Their activity increases with a fall in pH or P_{O_2} or an elevation in P_{CO_2} and their activity decreases if the opposite occurs. Peripheral chemoreceptors are most sensitive to changes in arterial P_{CO_2}.

The relative levels of pH, P_{O_2}, and P_{CO_2} influence the sensitivity of peripheral chemoreceptors to pH, P_{O_2}, or P_{CO_2}. When the P_{O_2} or pH is low, the carotid body sensitivity to P_{CO_2} is increased. Similarly, the carotid body sensitivity to oxygen is increased if the P_{CO_2} is elevated. However, under some circumstances these interactions can be antagonistic. At high altitude P_{O_2} falls because of the fall in atmospheric pressure. This stimulates ventilation but also reduces arterial

P_{CO_2} as carbon dioxide is blown off. The fall in P_{CO_2} reduces the primary drive for ventilation and the sensitivity of the carotid body chemoreceptors to arterial oxygen. This leads to a further fall in arterial P_{O_2}, enhancing oxygen's stimulatory effect on ventilation. Ultimately, a steady state is reached between the stimulatory response to *hypoxia* (low oxygen) and the inhibitory effect of *hypocapnia* (low CO_2).

ROLE OF THE LUNGS IN REGULATION OF ACID-BASE BALANCE
Ventilatory Response to Acid-Base Changes

* Because the CO_2–bicarbonate buffer system plays a significant role in regulating pH, the lungs can alter arterial pH by changing arterial P_{CO_2}.
* Ventilation is increased in response to metabolic acidemia.
* Ventilation is decreased in response to metabolic alkalemia.

Changes in ventilation affect the CO_2–bicarbonate buffer system and, therefore, the pH of arterial blood. The CO_2–bicarbonate buffer system is the major way in which the body maintains arterial pH because the lungs regulate the CO_2 level of the blood and the kidneys regulate the amount of bicarbonate (see chapter 4).

Carbon dioxide undergoes the following reaction in blood:

$$CO_2 + H_2O \Leftrightarrow H_2CO_3 \Leftrightarrow H^+ + HCO_3^- \qquad \text{(reaction 1)}$$

Using the Henderson-Hasselbalch equation, this reaction can be expressed in the following form:

$$pH = 6.1 + \log([HCO_3^-] / P_{CO_2})$$

Normal blood values can be substituted for the various parameters. To convert the units of mm Hg for P_{CO_2} to mEq/L, P_{CO_2} is multiplied by 0.03.

$$7.4 = 6.1 + \log (24 \text{ mEq/L}/(0.03 \times 40 \text{ mm Hg})) = 6.1 + \log 20/1$$

This relationship shows that as long as the ratio of bicarbonate to CO_2 is 20:1, pH will be 7.4. The body adjusts the amounts of these two substances in order to maintain a normal pH. The lungs regulate the amount of carbon dioxide.

Arterial hydrogen ion concentration can change for a variety of reasons. If the cause does not involve the lungs, it is said to be of *metabolic* origin. It is called *metabolic acidosis* if the pH decreases and *metabolic alkalosis* if the pH increases. If the lungs are the cause of the acid-base disturbance, the processes are called *respiratory acidosis* and *respiratory alkalosis*.

When the hydrogen ion concentration of the blood increases *(acidemia)* because of metabolic acidosis, the P_{CO_2} will also increase because (reaction 1) will be driven to the left. As described above, an elevation in arterial hydrogen ion concentration and P_{CO_2} will stimulate ventilation. The increase in ventilation will lower the P_{CO_2} driving (reaction 1) further to the left helping to lower the hydrogen ion concentration. In addition, the kidneys will generate bicarbonate and secrete hydrogen ions (see chapter 4).

In a similar manner, if arterial hydrogen ion concentration decreases *(alkalemia)* because of metabolic alkalosis, the low arterial hydrogen ion concentration will drive (reaction 1) to the right lowering the P_{CO_2}. The reduced arterial P_{CO_2} and hydrogen ion concentration will lower the ventilatory drive allowing P_{CO_2} to accumulate. This will generate additional hydrogen ions and help to return the pH to normal.

Altered Ventilation Causes Acid-Base Changes

> • An inability of the lungs to remove CO_2 results in respiratory acidemia.
> • Inappropriate removal of CO_2 by the lungs results in respiratory alkalemia.

Just as the lungs help to compensate for an acid-base imbalance, they can also cause acid-base imbalances. An inability of the lungs to remove CO_2 will lead to an elevation of arterial P_{CO_2} and acidemia. This is because the elevated P_{CO_2} leads to an increase in acid production as described in (reaction 1) above. In a similar manner, inappropriate removal of CO_2 will lower arterial P_{CO_2} and cause alkalemia.

· C H A P T E R · 6 ·

GASTROINTESTINAL PHYSIOLOGY

·

GENERAL ORGANIZATION
Components

- Gastrointestinal tract consists of 4 anatomical divisions: esophagus, stomach, small intestine, and colon or large intestine.
- Pancreas and liver play critical roles in digestion and absorption.

The gastrointestinal (GI) tract consists of 4 anatomical divisions that are the *esophagus, stomach, small intestine,* and *colon or large intestine.* The small intestine is subdivided into three sequential segments called the *duodenum, jejunum,* and *ileum.* The colon is subdivided into the *cecum;* the *ascending, transverse, descending,* and *sigmoid colons;* the *rectum*; and the *anal canal.*

Secretions from the pancreas, liver, and gallbladder play critical roles in the digestion and absorption of food. The pancreas secretes essential enzymes into the duodenum for the breakdown of ingested food as well as bicarbonate to neutralize stomach acid. The liver secretes bile salts essential for the absorption of fats, which are stored in the gallbladder for release into the duodenum.

Blood Supply

- GI tract is supplied by the splanchnic circulation.
- Portal system delivers all venous blood from the GI tract to the liver.

The splanchnic circulation supplies the GI tract as well as the pancreas, spleen, and liver. All venous blood leaving the GI tract travels through the portal vein to the liver. Here it passes through a second capillary bed where phagocytic *reticuloendothelial cells* clean the blood of any bacteria and other particles before the blood enters the general circulation. Most of the water-soluble, nonfat substances absorbed by the GI tract are also carried in the portal circulation to the liver. Liver cells remove about one third to one half of all nutrients. Fat-soluble substances absorbed by the GI tract are delivered to the circulation by the intestinal lymphatics.

Control and Coordination

GI function is controlled through a complex of sensors and effectors that coordinate motility and secretion so that digestion and absorption are optimized.

Coordination of GI function occurs through a complex of sensors and effectors. The movement of material from one GI section to the next must be coordinated with secretion from not only the GI tract but also the pancreas and gallbladder so that digestion and absorption of food is optimized. To accomplish this, receptors located both outside and inside the GI tract receive visual, mechanical, and chemical stimuli. Receptor activation induces responses through changes in the activity of the autonomic and enteric nervous systems as well as through the effect of hormones released from cells within the GI tract. A full appreciation of GI function requires an understanding of many interrelated reflex loops.

NEURAL AND CHEMICAL CONTROL
General Organization

- Motor activity of the GI tract is performed primarily by smooth muscle.
- The wall of the GI tract is multilayered consisting of glands, nerves, and muscles.
- The GI tract has its own nerve network called the enteric nervous system.

The musculature of the gastrointestinal (GI) tract is primarily smooth muscle. Only the upper half of the esophagus and the external anal sphincter are composed of skeletal muscle. Smooth muscle cells of the GI tract are electrically coupled like cardiac cells so that electrical activity is transmitted between cells. In the stomach and intestine, smooth muscle cells undergo spontaneous, rhythmic membrane depolarizations called the *basic electrical rhythm (BER)*. If these depolarizations are large enough, an action potential will be generated in the smooth muscle cell and a contraction will occur. As will be described later, neural and hormonal factors do not modify the BER but rather the smooth muscle cells, altering their likelihood of generating action potentials in response to the BER.

The wall of the GI tract is a multilayered structure (see Figure 6–1). The extent of each layer and its specific characteristics vary down the length of the gut. The names of the layers from the outer to the inner are: *serosa, longitudinal smooth muscle, myenteric plexus* (or *Auerbach's plexus*), *circular smooth muscle, submucosal plexus* (or *Meissner's plexus*), *submucosa*, and *mucosa*. The serosa and submucosa layers are composed of connective tissue. The two smooth muscle layers are oriented in different directions to enable the gut to shorten (longitudinal layer) or to constrict (circular layer), allowing the contents to be mixed and propelled in one direction. The submucosal and myenteric plexuses are neural networks that form the *enteric nervous system*. Extrinsic nerves and hormones influence the activity of the enteric nervous system. The mucosa layer

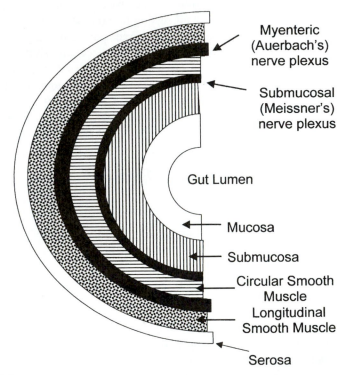

Figure 6–1
The wall of the gastrointestinal tract is composed of concentric layers of tissue that serve different functions.

is further subdivided into three layers. The *muscularis mucosa* is a thin muscle layer consisting of circularly and longitudinally oriented smooth muscle cells that sits atop the submucosa. Next is the *lamina propria*, which is composed of blood vessels, lymph glands, and connective tissue. The inner most layer is composed of *epithelial cells* that are specialized to secrete fluids, electrolytes, enzymes, or mucus into the lumen or are specialized for absorption of nutrients from the lumen.

The enteric nervous system performs both efferent and afferent functions (see Figure 6–2). The myenteric plexus primarily carries motor nerve activity to smooth muscle cells of the longitudinal and circular layers, while the submucosal plexus primarily carries nerve activity to the epithelial cells of the mucosal layer. In addition, these nerve layers receive sensory input from mechanoreceptors within the muscle layers and send this afferent information via the vagus and splanchnic nerves to the brain. Nerve cells within the myenteric and submucosal plexuses communicate with each other up and down the gut as well as between

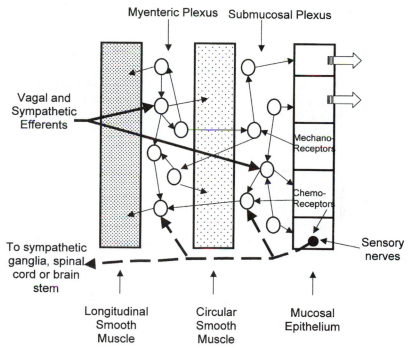

Figure 6–2
The wall of the gastrointestinal tract is innervated by an enteric nervous system (myenteric plexus and submucosal plexus) as well as by both branches of the autonomic nervous system (vagal and sympathetic efferents). In addition, sensory cells within the gut wall detect mechanical and chemical changes and send this information back to the spinal cord and brain.

the two plexuses. This permits reflex coordination of a variety of motor activities within the GI tract.

Neural Control

> • Sympathetic and parasympathetic nerves synapse with nerve cell bodies of the enteric nervous system.
> • Enteric nervous system releases a variety of neurotransmitters.

Both the sympathetic and parasympathetic nervous systems innervate the gut (see Figure 6–2). Sympathetic postganglionic nerve fibers end on nerve cell bodies within the enteric nervous system as well as on glands in the mucosa and smooth muscle cells of the circular muscle layer. Parasympathetic preganglionic nerves (primarily the vagus nerve) end on nerve cells of the myenteric and submucosal plexuses forming ganglia. The parasympathetic postganglionic nerves leave these ganglia and innervate glands within the mucosa and smooth muscle cells of the longitudinal muscle layer. Sympathetic nerves exert their effect through the release of the neural transmitter norepinephrine, which is generally inhibitory, while the parasympathetic nerves exert their effect through the release of acetylcholine, which is generally excitatory.

The enteric nervous system releases a variety of neurotransmitters. These transmitters include acetylcholine, nitric oxide, vasoactive intestinal peptide (VIP), enkephalins, serotonin, and substance P. The exact role and interaction of each of these chemical mediators is still being resolved.

Chemical Control

> • Numerous peptides regulate GI function.
> • GI peptides can be divided into three classes based on their site of release and action: hormones, paracrines, and neurocrines.
> • Hormones include secretin, gastrin, cholecystokinin (CCK), gastrin inhibitory peptide (GIP), and motilin.
> • Paracrines include somatostatin and histamine.
> • Neurocrines include vasoactive intestinal peptide (VIP), gastrin-releasing peptide (GRP), and enkephalins.

The peptides (short amino acid sequences) that act to regulate GI function are grouped into three classes: hormones, paracrines, and neurocrines. The physical relationship between the site of release and action distinguishes these classes. Peptide hormones are released by cells distant from their site of action and are carried to their target cells by the blood. In contrast, paracrine peptides are released by cells adjacent to their target cell and reach the target cell by diffusion. Neurocrine peptides are similar to paracrine peptides except that they are released solely by nerve cells.

Table 6–1 lists the action, site of release, and stimulus for each of the major GI regulatory peptides.

Reflex Control of Motility

- Reflexes exist within the gut to regulate motility.
- Mechanical and chemical stimuli initiate the various reflexes.
- Reflexes are classified in terms of the neural systems involved:
  —Those mediated solely by the enteric nervous system
  —Those that involve the prevertebral ganglia with sympathetic afferents and efferents
  —Those that involve the spinal cord and brain stem with vagal afferents and efferents
  —Those that involve a combination of the previous three.

The anatomical organization of the enteric and extrinsic nervous systems permits the existence of reflex loops within the gut. Distention in one part of the gut will result in relaxation in another part, for example. Or the release of a chemical substance in one segment will elicit a change in mechanical activity in another segment. These reflexes enable signals to be transmitted the length of the gut ensuring the coordinated movement of material from one end to the other.

Reflexes may be mediated solely through the enteric nervous system or involve nerve pathways that leave and return to the gut (sympathetic and parasympathetic). Those that leave the gut are divided into two groups. One group includes reflexes whose afferent nerves travel to the sympathetic prevertebral ganglia before returning via sympathetic efferents. The second group of reflexes includes those whose afferents travel to the spinal cord or the brain stem and then back via the vagus nerve. Characteristics of major GI reflexes are listed in Table 6–2.

MOTILITY

Chewing and Swallowing

- Chewing is important because
  —The food is lubricated by being mixed with saliva
  —The food is exposed to salivary amylase enzyme, which begins digestion
  —It breaks the food into small pieces.
- Swallowing is under the control of extrinsic nerves and the swallowing center.

TABLE 6–1   REGULATORY PEPTIDES OF THE GI TRACT

PEPTIDE	ACTION	SITE OF RELEASE	STIMULI
Hormones			
Gastrin	Stimulates acid secretion and growth of oxyntic gland mucosa	G cells of antrum	Peptides, amino acids, distention, vagal stimulation
CCK	Stimulates gallbladder contraction, pancreatic secretion, and growth of exocrine pancreas; inhibits gastric emptying	I cells of duodenum and jejunum	Peptides, amino acids, fatty acids
Secretin	Stimulates pancreatic and biliary bicarbonate secretion, gastric pepsinogen secretion, and growth of exocrine pancreas	S cells of duodenum	Acid
GIP	Stimulates insulin release and inhibits gastric acid secretion	Duodenum and jejunum	Glucose, amino acids, fatty acids
Motilin	Stimulates gastric and intestinal motility	Duodenum and jejunum	Nerves, fat, acid
Paracrines			
Somatostatin	Inhibits release of gastrin and other peptides; inhibits acid secretion	GI mucosa and pancreatic islets	Acid
Histamine	Stimulates gastric acid secretion	Oxyntic gland mucosa, ECL cell	Gastrin
Neurocrines			
VIP	Relaxes sphincters, gut circular muscle; stimulates intestinal and pancreatic secretion	Mucosa and smooth muscle	Nerve activity
GRP	Stimulates gastrin release	Gastric mucosa	Nerve activity
Enkephalins	Stimulates smooth muscle contraction and inhibits intestinal secretion	Mucosa and smooth muscle	Nerve activity

This table groups the peptides involved in influencing GI functioning based on whether they are hormones, paracrines, or neurocrines. The physiological action of each peptide is listed along with its site of release and the primary stimulus responsible for its release.

TABLE 6–2 NEURALLY MEDIATED REFLEXES OF THE GI TRACT THAT CONTROL MOTILITY

REFLEX	ORIGIN	STIMULUS	EFFECTOR SITE	EFFECT	PATHWAY
Gastrocolic	Stomach	Distention	Colon	Increased motility	Prevertebral gang & symp
Gastroileal (or gastroenteric)	Stomach	Distention	Ileum	Increased motility	Brain stem & vagus plus enteric
Vagovagal	Stomach	Distention	Stomach	Decreased motility	Brain stem & vagus
Enterogastric	Small intestine; colon	Distention; acid; osmolarity; protein; fat	Stomach	Inhibit motility	Prevertebral gang & symp plus enteric
Intestinointestinal	Small intestine	Distention	Small intestine	Decreased motility	Prevertebral gang & symp
Peristaltic	Small intestine	Distention	Small intestine	Increased & decreased motility	Enteric & extrinsic
Duodenocolic	Duodenum	Distention	Colon	Increased motility	Prevertebral gang & symp
Colonoileal	Colon	Distention	Ileum	Decreased motility	Prevertebral gang & symp
Peritoneointestinal	Peritoneum	Pain	Intestine	Decreased motility	Prevertebral gang & symp
Renointestinal	Kidney	Pain	Intestine	Decreased motility	Prevertebral gang & symp
Vesicointestinal	Bladder	Pain	Intestine	Decreased motility	Prevertebral gang & symp
Somatointestinal	Skin	Pain	Intestine	Decreased motility	Prevertebral gang & symp
Defecation	Rectum	Distention	Internal anal sphincter, rectum	Sphincter relaxation; increased rectum motility	Enteric

This table describes five characteristics of major reflexes in the GI tract. "Origin" refers to the segment of the gut where the reflex originates, that is, where the sensor is located. "Stimulus" refers to what is sensed and initiates the reflex. "Effector Site" refers to the portion of the gut that is acted upon by the reflex and "Effect" refers to the response of the Effector Site. "Pathway" refers to the proposed neural pathway involved. Note that some reflexes make use of more than one pathway. "Gang" = ganglion; "symp" = sympathetic.

Chewing of food serves three purposes: (1) Chewing mixes food with saliva, lubricating it and making it easier to swallow. (2) Chewing mixes food with salivary amylase, beginning the digestive process because amylase breaks down starch. (3) Chewing breaks food into small pieces to facilitate swallowing.

The muscles of the pharynx involved in swallowing are striated muscles and are controlled by extrinsic nerves. Receptors in the pharynx sense the presence of food particles and send signals to the swallowing center in the brain stem. This initiates rhythmic firing of neurons in the center, which sends stimulatory signals to the striated muscle producing a rhythmic contraction. This propels food toward the esophagus.

Esophagus

- The esophagus prevents air from entering the GI tract through the function of the upper esophageal sphincter.
- The esophagus prevents GI contents from re-entering the esophagus from the stomach through the function of the lower esophageal sphincter.
- The contraction that sweeps down the esophagus is the result of intrinsic and extrinsic stimuli.
- Achalasia is a condition in which the lower esophageal sphincter does not open, causing food to accumulate in the esophagus.

The upper and lower esophageal sphincters prevent air from entering the GI tract and prevent gastric contents from entering the esophagus.

To move the swallowed food down the esophagus, a pressure wave has to be generated by the contracting striated and smooth muscles. This wave of contraction or *primary peristaltic contraction* begins just below the upper esophageal sphincter and travels down the length of the esophagus. The primary peristaltic contraction is initiated by the rhythmic firing of nerves from the swallowing center, but in the absence of extrinsic innervation, the enteric nervous system and smooth muscle cells can generate the peristaltic contraction. If the primary peristaltic contraction is insufficient to empty the esophagus, one or more *secondary peristaltic* contractions are initiated locally. As these contractions propel the food toward the lower esophageal sphincter, the smooth muscle of the sphincter relaxes to allow the food to pass and then contracts again. Sphincter relaxation is mediated through the vagus nerve but the transmitter has not conclusively been identified (VIP and/or nitric oxide). If the sphincter does not open properly, the condition of *achalasia* develops and food accumulates in the esophagus.

Stomach

- In terms of motility the stomach is divided into orad (proximal) and caudad (distal) areas.
- Orad area is thin walled, holds large volumes of food because of receptive relaxation, and contracts weakly and infrequently.
- Caudad area is thick walled with strong and frequent contractions that mix and propel food into the duodenum.
- Contractions of the caudad stomach
  —Are different during interdigestive and digestive periods
  —Originate from BER of smooth muscle cells during the digestive period
  —Are modified by extrinsic nerves and hormones, which are regulated in turn by stomach contents.

The stomach is divided into the orad and caudad areas based on muscularity and contractile force and pattern. The esophagus empties into the orad stomach. This portion of the stomach is thin walled with weak infrequent contractions. Its primary function is to store food. Through a vagovagal reflex initiated by swallowing or distention of the stomach, smooth muscle of the orad stomach undergoes *receptive relaxation* to accommodate the incoming food. Cutting the vagus prevents receptive relaxation and the hormone cholecystokinin (CCK) enhances receptive relaxation. Because of receptive relaxation the orad stomach can contain as much as 1500 mL of food. Little mixing occurs in the orad stomach because the contractions are weak and infrequent, so the ingested food remains in unmixed layers.

In contrast, the caudad stomach has well-developed muscle layers and produces strong contractions. In the interdigestive period when the stomach is empty, every 90 minutes a strong contraction, the *migrating motor complex (MMC)*, passes though the caudad stomach and into the intestine. The MMC sweeps any remaining particles from the stomach into the duodenum and is thought to have a "house cleaning" function. The MMC is initiated by the cyclical release of the hormone *motilin* from the small intestine and is inhibited by food in the stomach. It is not known how the cyclical release of motilin is produced.

During the digestive phase, the frequency and magnitude of contractions within the caudad stomach increase. The objective of these contractions is to mix the stomach contents with enzymes and acid, break the food into small particles, and propel the contents into the small intestine at a rate that is consistent with optimal digestion and absorption. Therefore, coordination between stomach and intestine is critical. The rate of stomach emptying is regulated by receptors in the stomach and intestine that sense different properties of the foodstuff (see Gastroileal and Enterogastric reflexes in Table 6–2). Stomach receptors sense the physical characteristics of the material such as volume and particle size. These stimuli alter emptying primarily through the intrinsic properties of the gut smooth muscle cells themselves. Intestinal receptors sense chemical characteristic such as osmolarity, pH, and lipid content although duodenal volume also influences stomach emptying. These stimuli alter emptying through mechanisms that involve nerves and hormones. The *basic electrical rhythm (BER)* of smooth muscle cells form the basis of stomach contractions. The ability of BER to induce smooth muscle contraction is altered by the activity of extrinsic nerves and hormones, brought into play by stomach and intestine receptors. Large stomach volumes empty faster than small volumes. Liquids empty faster than solids, and solids must be reduced to particles less than 2 mm^3 to empty rapidly. The presence of calories, in the form of fats or acid, slows emptying. Fat in the duodenum stimulates the release of CCK from I cells of the duodenum, which increases contraction of the caudad stomach while at the same time enhancing reflexive relaxation of the orad stomach causing the net movement of food toward the orad stomach. Acid in the duodenum inhibits caudad stomach contraction through neural mechanisms that involve the enteric nervous system. Other hormones like gastrin inhibitory peptide (GIP) and secretin have been shown to inhibit stomach emptying but only at nonphysiological concentrations.

Small Intestine

> • Motility of the small intestine serves four purposes:
>   —Mixing contents with enzymes and other secretions
>   —Further reduction in particle size
>   —Maximizing exposure of the contents to membranes of intestinal cells for absorption and digestion
>   —Propulsion of contents into the large intestine.
> • Two basic motility patterns exist: segmentation and peristalsis.
> • Response of smooth muscle to the basic electrical rhythm is modified by extrinsic nerves and hormones responding to changes in intestinal volume and contents to produce appropriate motility patterns.
> • Several reflex responses help coordinate motility patterns: (1) peristaltic reflex, (2) intestinointestinal reflex, (3) gastroileal reflex, (4) enterogastric reflex, and (5) duodenocolic reflex.

Motility in the small intestine ensures that the contents are well mixed with enzymes and other secretions present in the intestine, further broken down into smaller particles, brought into close contact with the cells lining the intestine to maximize absorption and digestion, and moved into the large intestine. These functions are accomplished by two basic motility patterns: segmentation and propulsion. During *segmentation*, contraction of short lengths (1–5 cm) of intestine occurs, but they are not coordinated with adjacent segments. This causes the contents to be divided and forced in both the orad and caudad directions. When the contracted segment relaxes again, material from adjacent segments flows back into the relaxing segment and no net movement down the length of the intestine occurs. During *peristalsis,* however, there is a coordination of contraction-relaxation in the orad to caudad direction. This results in the net movement of the contents in the caudad direction. What determines the type of motility pattern that occurs at any particular moment has not been determined; however, the volume and nature of the intestinal contents influence the pattern.

As in the stomach, the smooth muscle basic electrical rhythm is influenced by nerve activity and hormones, which enhance or reduce the ability of the BER to stimulate smooth muscle contraction. When the intestine is empty as during the interdigestive period, a migrating motor complex sweeps from the stomach along the small intestine every 90 minutes in response to cyclical changes in motilin concentration in the blood. During a meal, however, the contractile activity of the small intestine increases and both segmentation and peristalsis are evident.

As before, parasympathetic nerve stimulation increases contraction while sympathetic nerve stimulation reduces contraction. The neural mediators for these effects are incompletely understood, but vasoactive intestinal peptide (VIP) and nitric oxide have been shown to inhibit contraction and serotonin and opioid peptides stimulate contraction. Hormones such as gastrin, CCK, serotonin, and insulin stimulate contraction while secretin and glucagon inhibit it, but their physiological role is unclear.

Several reflexes help coordinate the contractile activity along the length of the small intestine. In general terms, the reflexes help to move food along the intestine, to meter the amount of food entering from the stomach, and to move food into the colon as more enters the duodenum. The *peristaltic reflex* helps propel food along the intestine. Distention of one segment of the small intestine reflexively induces contraction above and relaxation below the distention resulting in a peristaltic pattern of contraction. This peristaltic reflex involves both extrinsic and enteric nerves. The *intestinointestinal reflex* prevents further movement of food into an already distended portion of the small intestine by blocking intestinal contractions. This reflex depends solely on extrinsic nerves. The *gastroileal reflex (or gastroenteric reflex)* is characterized by increased contraction of the ileum in association with contraction and secretion of the stomach. The effect is to move ileal contents into the large intestine. The *enterogastric reflex* inhibits gastric emptying in response to food in the small intestine (or colon). This reflex is initiated by distention, osmolarity, acidity, and protein and is mediated through both enteric and extrinsic nerves. The *duodenocolic reflex* stimulates contraction of the colon in response to food in the duodenum. This ensures that the colon is ready to receive additional food from the small intestine. It is initiated by distention and mediated through the extrinsic nervous system.

Vomiting

> • Vomiting is the reflex contraction of both the stomach and small intestine
>   to rid the body of noxious or toxic substances.
> • It is controlled by the vomiting center in the brain.

Vomiting is the body's way of removing noxious or toxic substances from the GI
tract; however, it can also occur in response to a wide variety of other stimuli that
are not chemical such as dizziness, tickling in the back of the throat, or painful
injury.

   Vomiting is controlled by the vomiting center in the medulla. This center
receives afferent information from a variety of receptors throughout the body.
Vomiting involves the coordinated contraction of the skeletal muscle of the abdominal wall and diaphragm along with the smooth muscle of the esophagus,
stomach, and small intestine. It begins with contraction of the stomach and
small intestine producing a reverse peristalsis. These contractions build and are
combined with skeletal muscle contractions to expel the food out of the mouth.

Large Intestine or Colon

> • There are two basic motility patterns: segmentation and mass movement.
> • Motility regulated primarily by enteric nervous system.
> • Defecation involves voluntary and involuntary reflexes.

The large intestine has two primary motility patterns: segmentation and mass
movement. As in other segments of the GI tract, *segmentation* in the large intestine causes the contents to be continuously mixed so that they are exposed to the
gut epithelium enabling effective absorption of water and electrolytes. Segmentation does not move the intestinal contents toward the rectum. Segmentation
causes the large intestine to appear divided into small, interconnected sacs called
haustra.

   One to three times a day a coordinated peristaltic contraction occurs called a
mass movement that propels the contents of one segment of the large intestine
into the next downstream segment. Segmentation stops in the area of the large
intestine undergoing the mass movement and the haustra disappear giving this
portion of the large intestine a smooth surface. Both segmentation and mass
movement are under enteric nervous system control because they occur in the absence of extrinsic nerves.

   Defecation involves both voluntary and involuntary reflexes. Mass movement propels material from the sigmoid colon into the rectum. Distention of the

rectum by this material initiates an involuntary relaxation of the smooth muscle of internal anal sphincter called the *rectosphincteric reflex* (or *defecation reflex*) as well as a peristaltic contraction of the rectum. This reflex is mediated through the enteric nervous system as well as parasympathetic nerves from the pelvic portion of the spinal cord. The contraction of the rectum signals the urge to defecate. If this is convenient, then the external anal sphincter is relaxed by voluntary inhibition of motor nerves to the skeletal muscle of the external anal sphincter. If inconvenient, relaxation is not initiated, the rectum accommodates to the increased volume reducing the intensity of the rectosphincteric reflex, and the internal anal sphincter contracts.

SECRETION
General Principles

- GI secretions function to lubricate, protect, sterilize, neutralize, and digest.
- Secretions arise from specialized cells lining the GI tract, the pancreas, liver, and gallbladder.
- Secretions are generated by clusters of cells connected to the lumen of the GI tract by ducts whose cells modify the fluid as it passes by.
- Secretion rate and composition are regulated by autonomic nerves and hormones.

The secretions of the GI tract serve many functions. Some (water and mucus) act as lubricants to ease the passage of food. Some protect the cells lining the gut by forming an impenetrable barrier (mucus), while others can be caustic to organisms such as bacteria thereby helping to sterilize ingested food (hydrochloride (HCl)). Also, secretions (HCO_3) neutralize the luminal contents so that the pH is optimal for the proper functioning of digestive enzymes. Finally, secretions contain enzymes needed for the breakdown of fats, carbohydrates, and proteins.

In the salivary glands and pancreas, secretions are formed by grapelike clusters of cells *(acinar cells)* located at the ends of ducts that lead to the lumen of the GI tract (see Figure 6–3). Because of this arrangement, the composition of the primary secretion can be adjusted as it flows along the duct. In the stomach, the organization is more complicated in that multiple cell types secreting different substances (mucus, HCl, enzymes) communicate with a common duct leading to the stomach lumen.

The autonomic nervous system and hormones influence the composition and rate of secretion. Reflex communication between gut segments ensures that secretions are of appropriate volume and composition for optimal digestion.

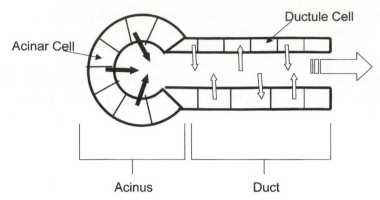

Figure 6–3
The salivary gland is composed of acinar and ductule cells.

Salivary Secretion

- Secretions serve digestive (amylase, lipase), lubricative (mucus), and protective functions.
- The three paired salivary glands are the parotid, submaxillary, and sublingual.
- Glands are composed of acinar cells that secrete an isotonic fluid and ductule cells that reabsorb Na and Cl ions and secrete K and HCO_3 ions.
- Salivary concentrations of K and HCO_3 ions are higher while those of Na and Cl ions are less than in blood.
- Saliva is hypotonic to plasma except at maximum secretory rates when it becomes isotonic.
- Glands are under the control of the autonomic nervous system where both branches stimulate secretion

Salivary secretion serves digestive, lubricative, and protective functions. Saliva contains two digestive enzymes, alpha amylase and lingual lipase. *Alpha amylase* is responsible for digesting starch and remains active into the caudad stomach where it is inactivated by the high acidity. *Lingual lipase* begins the digestion of triglycerides and because it is not inactivated by the acidity of the stomach, remains active into the duodenum. The mucus content of the saliva helps to lubricate the swallowed food. Saliva also protects by diluting and buffering potentially harmful constituents of food as well as by washing and dissolving food particles from between the teeth. Finally, it contains a number of substances that kill bacteria.

There are three paired salivary glands, the *parotid, submaxillary,* and *sublingual,* each composed of *acinar* and *ductule* cells. Acinar cells form blind sacs that are connected to the mouth by ducts. Ductule cells are of two types: *intercalated* and *striated.* Acinar cells are responsible for forming saliva while ductule cells modify the composition of the saliva.

    Acinar cells are functionally polar in that the permeability properties of the basolateral cell membrane are different than those of the luminal cell membrane (see Figure 6–4). A similar polarity is seen in kidney tubule epithelial cells

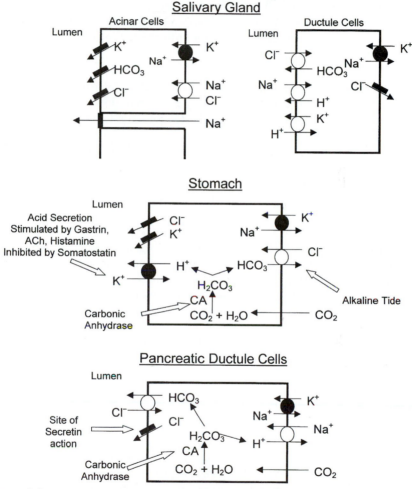

Figure 6–4
Secretory cells in the gastrointestinal tract utilize a variety of transport mechanisms to produce the fluid that they release. The transport mechanisms for the salivary gland, stomach, and pancreas are diagramed in this figure. Notice that most couple the movement of Na into the cell down the concentration gradient generated by the Na-K ATPase to move other molecules (eg, Cl^-, H^+).

making the ion transport processes of the salivary glands and kidney tubules very similar. The activity of the Na-K ion pump in the basolateral membrane drives the process by generating a concentration gradient favoring the diffusion of Na ions into the acinar cell. This movement of Na into the cells drives the inward movement of Cl ions by a cotransport process and produces an elevated intracellular chloride ion concentration. Chloride ions then diffuse down their concentration gradient through ion-specific channels in the luminal cell membrane. In this way Cl ions are secreted by the acinar cells through a secondary active transport process dependent upon the activity of the Na-K ion pump. Sodium ions follow Cl ions to maintain electrical neutrality by diffusing between the acinar cells. K and HCO_3 ions are secreted into the lumen by passive diffusion through ion channels. As a result of this net movement of ions from the basolateral to the luminal side of acinar cells, water follows. The net effect is that acinar cells produce a fluid that is isotonic to blood but whose concentration of Na and Cl ions is less than that of blood and whose K and HCO_3 concentration is greater than that of blood.

As saliva flows along the duct to the mouth, ductule cells modify the composition (see Figure 6–4). The luminal membrane of ductule cells reabsorbs Na ions and secretes K ions through H ion counter transport processes that are both dependent upon the activity of the Na-K ion pump in the basolateral membrane. The Na-K ion pump maintains a low intracellular Na concentration and an elevated K ion concentration favoring their movement into and out of the cell, respectively, in exchange for H ions. In addition, ductule cells reabsorb Cl and secrete HCO_3 ions through a counter transport system located in the luminal cell membrane. The net effect of these ion movements is to lower the Na and Cl ion concentrations and to raise the K and HCO_3 ion concentrations of the saliva. Ductule cells reabsorb more ions than they secrete and because they are impermeable to water, the fluid becomes hypotonic. The impact of ductule cells on salivary composition depends upon how long they are in contact with the saliva. The faster the rate of salivary secretion, the less effect they have and the more the final composition of the saliva matches that produced by the acinar cells. For example, at maximum salivary flow, saliva is isotonic and contains more Na and Cl ions than at a slower rate.

The rate of salivary secretion is regulated by the activity of both the sympathetic and parasympathetic nervous systems. Increased activity of either increases the rate of secretion, although parasympathetic nerve activity has a greater effect on secretion rate. Acetylcholine and norepinephrine released from parasympathetic and sympathetic postganglionic nerves, respectively, increase secretion by (1) increasing the activity of the ion transport systems, (2) increasing blood flow to the salivary glands, (3) increasing the metabolism of the cells, and (4) causing contraction of *myoepithelial cells* surrounding the acinar cells causing saliva to be forced from the glands. Sustained autonomic nerve activity will also cause growth of salivary glands. Chewing, taste, and smell increase nerve activity and secretion while sleep, fear, and fatigue reduce nerve activity and secretion.

Gastric Secretion

Formation

> - Gastric secretion has four components: hydrochloric acid, pepsin, mucus, and intrinsic factor.
> - The stomach is divided into oxyntic gland and pyloric gland areas based on secretory function.
> - The oxyntic gland area comprises: (1) parietal or oxyntic cells that secrete acid and intrinsic factor, and (2) chief or peptic cells that secrete pepsinogen and gastric lipase.
> - The pyloric gland area is composed of G cells that secrete gastrin and mucus-secreting cells.
> - The H-K ion ATPase of parietal cells is responsible for acid secretion.

Stomach secretions are composed of four substances: hydrochloric acid, *pepsin*, mucus and *intrinsic factor*. Hydrochloric acid is important because it kills bacteria contained within ingested food, begins the breakdown of proteins, and converts the inactive *pepsinogen* into the active enzyme pepsin, which breaks down protein. Mucus serves a lubricative role as well as a protective function against the caustic effects of the hydrochloric acid. Intrinsic factor is required for the absorption of vitamin B_{12} and is the only stomach secretion that is essential.

Distinct regions of the stomach produce these secretions. The proximal 80% of the stomach is called the *oxyntic gland area* and is composed two cell types: (1) *parietal* (or *oxyntic*) cells and (2) *chief* (or *peptic*) cells. The remainder of the stomach is called the *pyloric gland area* (or *antrum*) and is made up of three cell types: (1) *G (gastrin) cells,* 2) *mucus cells,* and (3) *D cells.* The cell types in each area and their secretions are listed in Table 6–3.

In the oxyntic gland, parietal and chief cells are arranged so that their secretions are released into a common duct that passes to the surface of the stomach. Unlike salivary secretion, gastric secretion remains isotonic to blood at all secretion rates; however, its ionic composition changes with rate. As secretion rate increases from a basal to a maximum rate, the amount of Na ions decreases and the amount of H ions increases. This change is explained in terms of a shift from a nonparietal to a parietal cell secretion. The nonparietal cell secretion contains primarily Na ions and is formed at a low rate. But as secretory rate increases, parietal cell secretion dominates and it contains primarily H ions.

The secretion of acid by parietal cells is the result of the action of an H-K ion ATPase pump located in the luminal membrane of these cells (see Figure 6–4).

TABLE 6–3 AREAS OF THE STOMACH, CELL TYPES IN EACH, AND THEIR SECRETIONS		
STOMACH REGIONS	**CELL TYPE**	**SECRETIONS**
Oxyntic gland area	Parietal (oxyntic) cells	Acid, instrinsic factor
	Chief (peptic) cells	Pepsinogen, gastric lipase
Pyloric gland area	G cells	Gastrin
(antrum)	Mucus cells	Mucus, pepsinogen
	D cells	Somatostatin

This table lists the stomach areas, the cell types present in each area, and the secretions of the cell types.

Hydrogen ions are moved out of the cell in exchange for K ions through an energy-dependent process. The hydrogen ions for secretion are formed from the conversion of CO_2 and H_2O to H and HCO_3 ions through the action of *carbonic anhydrase* within parietal cells. A similar process is involved in acid secretion by kidney epithelial cells. The bicarbonate formed is secreted on the basolateral side of the cell in exchange for Cl ions. During elevated acid secretion, as occurs during a meal, the bicarbonate concentration of venous blood leaving the stomach increases and is called the *alkaline tide*.

Regulation of Acid Secretion

- Acid secretion is controlled by gastrin, parasympathetic nerves, and histamine.
- Histamine is released from enterochromaffin-like cells (ECL) and potentiates the stimulatory effects of parasympathetic nerves and gastrin.
- Acid secretion is inhibited by somatostatin released from stomach cells and by the presence of digested food in the duodenum.
- Acid secretion is stimulated by signals from the mouth (cephalic phase), stomach (gastric phase) and intestine (intestinal phase).

Parietal cells contain receptors for gastrin, acetylcholine (ACh), and histamine, which, when stimulated by their specific agonists, stimulate acid secretion. Both acetylcholine and histamine, acting through their specific receptors, initiate a cascade of cellular events that result in protein phosphorylation and stimulation of H ion secretion. The mechanism by which gastrin stimulates acid secretion has not been delineated. The presence of any one of these agents enhances or potentiates the stimulatory effect of the other two. *Gastrin* is released from the G cells of the stomach, circulates in the blood, and acts on the parietal cells. *Acetylcholine* is released from vagal parasympathetic postganglionic nerves that end on parietal cells. *Histamine* is released from *enterochromaffin-like (ECL) cells* located within the gut mucosa by parasympathetic nerves (acetylcholine) and by gastrin.

Between meals, the interdigestive period, acid secretion is at a slow rate due to the action of *somatostatin* and the absence of stimulatory signals. In the interdigestive period, stomach fluid is acid, which stimulates the release of somatostatin from the stomach mucosa. Somatostatin directly inhibits acid secretion by parietal cells and indirectly by inhibiting gastrin release from G cells.

Acid secretion is divided into three phases based on the origin of the stimulatory signals. The *cephalic phase* includes stimuli initiated by the taste, smell, and sight of food. It is mediated solely by the vagus nerve through direct stimulation of parietal cells and through stimulating gastrin release. No food need actually be swallowed to initiate this phase of acid secretion. The *gastric phase* includes stimuli that depend upon the presence of food in the stomach. Food reduces the acidity of the stomach contents, which reduces somatostatin release and removes its inhibitory effect. Also, distention of the stomach through mechanoreceptors and the enteric nervous system directly activate parietal cells as well as stimulate gastrin release. Finally, digested protein stimulates gastrin release. The gastric phase is responsible for stimulating the majority (60%) of acid secretion. When protein metabolites reach the duodenum, they produce an additional stimulation of acid secretion known as the *intestinal phase*. This stimulation is the result of distention probably mediated through the action of an intestinal hormone, *enterooxyntin,* on parietal cells and the presence of absorbed amino acids stimulating parietal cells.

As food moves from the stomach into the small intestine, reflexes are initiated that inhibit gastric acid secretion. The removal of food from the stomach allows the acidity of the stomach fluid to increase, which initiates the inhibitory effects of somatostatin. In addition, the acidity, osmolarity, and fat content of the food in the duodenum initiate reflexes that reduce gastric acid secretion. The mediators and pathways of these have not been determined. The net effect is that acid secretion slowly returns to that during the interdigestive period.

Regulation of Pepsin Secretion

- Pepsinogen secretion regulated primarily by vagal nerve stimulation.
- Acid is important not only for pepsin formation but also for enhancing its secretion.

Acetylcholine, released from vagal postganglionic nerve fibers, is the primary stimulus for pepsinogen secretion by chief cells. Vagal stimulation of pepsinogen release occurs during both the cephalic and gastric phases. However, acid in the stomach is critical not only for the activation of pepsinogen as pepsin but also for its secretion. Acid triggers the enteric nerves to stimulate pepsinogen release by releasing acetylcholine. Secondly, acid in the duodenum stimulates the release of *secretin*, which stimulates pepsinogen release from chief cells. Because acid enhances pepsinogen release, the release is maximum only when there is sufficient acid present to activate the enzyme.

Regulation of Mucus Secretion

> • Soluble and insoluble mucus are secreted by cells of the stomach.
> • Vagal nerve stimulation increases the secretion of soluble mucus while chemicals and physical irritation stimulates the secretion of insoluble mucus.

Cells of the stomach wall secrete both soluble and insoluble mucus. Soluble mucus mixes with the contents of the stomach and helps to lubricate this material. Insoluble mucus forms a protective barrier against the high acidity of the stomach content. Because of these functions, secretion of both forms of mucus increase in association with a meal. Vagal nerve stimulation increases soluble mucus secretion while chemicals and physical stimuli increase the secretion of insoluble mucus.

Regulation of Intrinsic Factor Secretion

> • Secretion of intrinsic factor is essential for the absorption of vitamin B_{12} by the ileum.
> • Little is known about the regulation of intrinsic factor secretion.

Intrinsic factor is secreted by parietal cells of the stomach. It binds vitamin B_{12} present in ingested food, and the formation of this complex is crucial for absorption of the vitamin by the ileum. Without intrinsic factor, the vitamin cannot be absorbed. This is the only function of the stomach that is essential. Little is known about the regulation of intrinsic factor secretion.

Pancreatic Secretion

Formation

> • Secretion has aqueous and enzymatic components.
> • Enzymatic component is produced by acinar cells and is essential for the proper digestion and absorption of carbohydrates, fats, and proteins.
>
> *(continued)*

> (*continued*)
> - Aqueous component is produced by ductule cells and is important for neutralizing stomach acid in the duodenum so pancreatic enzymes can function properly.
> - Bicarbonate is secreted by ductule cells through a Cl-HCO_3 exchanger in the luminal membrane.

The pancreas is both an exocrine and an endocrine gland. In this section, the exocrine function of the pancreas will be described. The endocrine function is described in chapter 7, Endocrine Physiology. The pancreatic cells involved in exocrine secretion make up more than 80% of the organ's volume and produce over a liter of fluid each day.

The secretion of the exocrine pancreas has an enzymatic and aqueous component. The functional secretory unit is composed of acinar and ductule cells, which are organized as described for the salivary gland. However, in the pancreas these two cell types are responsible for specific components of the secretion. Acinar cells secrete the enzymatic component and ductule cells secrete the aqueous component. Ducts from clusters of acinar cells come together to form a single large pancreatic duct that empties into the proximal portion of the duodenum.

The enzyme secretions of the pancreatic acinar cells unlike those of the salivary gland are essential for complete digestion and absorption of ingested food. The secretion contains enzymes to digest carbohydrates (*pancreatic amylase*), fats (*pancreatic lipase, cholesterol esterase, phospholipase*), proteins (*trypsinogen, chymotrypsinogen, proelastase, procarboxypolypeptidase, proaminopeptidase*), and nucleic acids (*ribonuclease, deoxyribonuclease*). Synthesized enzymes are stored within the cell in *zymogen granules* located near the luminal side of the cell. Upon stimulation, the membranes of the granules fuse with the cell membrane and release their contents into the duct leading to the small intestine. The rate of secretion, but not the rate of synthesis, is regulated by nerves and hormones. All enzymes except the proteolytic enzymes (trypsinogen, chymotrypsinogen, proelastase, procarboxypolypeptidase, proaminopeptidase) are secreted in an active form. The proteolytic enzymes become activated in the lumen of the small intestine.

The ductule cells are responsible for secretion of the aqueous component of pancreatic secretion. As with gastric secretion, the composition of the fluid is the result of secretions from two different unidentified cell types. One cell type secretes an isotonic NaCl solution at a slow rate, which forms the basal aqueous secretion. Upon stimulation, a second cell type is activated, which secretes an isotonic bicarbonate-rich, chloride-deficient solution. The higher the secretion rate, the greater proportion comes from the second cell type and the more alkaline the secretion. Pancreatic bicarbonate secretion into the duodenum is critical for neutralizing the acidic material coming from the stomach thereby enabling the pancreatic enzymes to function properly.

Bicarbonate secretion involves ion exchangers that are similar to those involved with acid secretion in the stomach parietal cells except they are located on different membrane surfaces (see Figure 6–4). In pancreatic ductule cells, the luminal cell membrane contains a $Cl–HCO_3$ ion exchanger that is responsible for bicarbonate secretion. Bicarbonate is derived from the intracellular conversion of CO_2 and H_2O by carbonic anhydrase. The hydrogen ions that arise from this conversion are secreted on the basolateral side of the cell through a Na–H ion exchanger. This exchanger is driven by the influx of Na ions down a concentration gradient created by the action of the Na-K-ATPase in the basolateral cell membrane. For optimal bicarbonate ion secretion, the intracellular Cl ion concentration must be kept low. This occurs by the passive diffusion of Cl through a Cl ion specific channel in the luminal cell membrane. The rate of bicarbonate secretion is determined by the ability of Cl to move through this channel and is the site at which hormones, like *secretin*, stimulate bicarbonate secretion.

Regulation

- There is a cephalic, gastric, and intestinal phase to pancreatic secretion with the intestinal phase being the major stimulus.
- Cephalic and gastric phases stimulate the enzyme component of secretion through the action on acinar cells of acetylcholine released from vagal nerves.
- Intestinal phase is initiated by acid, protein, and fat in duodenal contents.
- Acid releases secretin, which is the primary stimulus of aqueous component; fat and protein release cholecystokinin (CCK), which stimulates enzymatic component; all three substances stimulate vagal nerve release of acetylcholine causing secretion of enzymatic component.

As with gastric secretion, the control of pancreatic secretion is divided into cephalic, gastric, and intestinal phases, with the intestinal phase being responsible for controlling over 70% of the secretory response.

In the cephalic phase, the site, smell, and taste of food initiates the enzymatic component of pancreatic secretion through the stimulation of acinar cells by acetylcholine released from vagal nerve endings. The distention of the stomach initiates the gastric phase, which also stimulates the enzymatic component of secretion through the acetylcholine-mediated action of the vagus nerve on acinar cells.

The intestinal phase of pancreatic secretion is initiated by the presence of acid, fat, and protein in the duodenum. Cells lining the proximal most portion of the duodenum are exposed to acidic material coming from the stomach. If the pH of this material is 4.5 or lower, the *S cells* in this portion of the duodenum release the hormone secretin. *Secretin* acts on pancreatic ductule cells to increase their rate of aqueous secretion, and this alkaline secretion neutralizes the acidity (see Figure 6–4). Secretin is the primary stimulus of the aqueous component. The presence of fat and protein digestion products in the duodenum is sensed by I cells and they secrete *cholecystokinin (CCK)*. CCK acts on pancreatic acinar cells to stimulate the enzymatic component of secretion. Acid, fat, and protein also stimulate the enzymatic component of secretion through a vagal reflex mediated by acetylcholine. Finally, CCK and acetylcholine increase the effectiveness of secretin.

Bile Secretion

Synthesis and Storage

- Bile is composed of bile acids, phospholipids, cholesterol, bile pigments, electrolytes, and water.
- In the small intestine bile emulsifies fats, forms micelles of lipid metabolites and complexes substances for excretion.
- The liver synthesizes new and recycles secreted bile acids through the enterohepatic circulation.
- The gallbladder stores and concentrates bile.

Bile is a mixture of *bile acids,* phospholipids, cholesterol, *bile pigments,* electrolytes, and water with bile acids comprising the largest proportion (approximately 50%). The components of bile are generated in the liver and stored in the gallbladder until release into the duodenum is initiated (see Figure 6–5). Bile acids and phospholipids are *amphipathic* molecules, which means that they have both water-soluble and water-insoluble portions. This enables them to dissolve fats in the watery mixture of the small intestine and to form aggregates of lipids called *micelles.* Both functions greatly facilitate the digestion and absorption of fats. Bile is also one way that the body has for excreting excess cholesterol. *Bile pigments* are primarily *bilirubin,* the metabolic end product of hemoglobin breakdown by macrophage in the reticuloendothelial system of the liver. The liver removes bilirubin from the blood and converts it into a soluble salt for excretion in the bile. Electrolytes, primarily bicarbonate ions, and water are added to bile in the liver and as it passes along the bile duct to the gallbladder (see Figure 6–5). The volume and bicarbonate content are under hormonal control.

Bile acids are synthesized and secreted by liver cells. Bile acids are modified cholesterol molecules in which one or more hydroxyl molecules have been removed. The liver synthesizes two bile acids, *chenodeoxycholic acid* and *cholic*

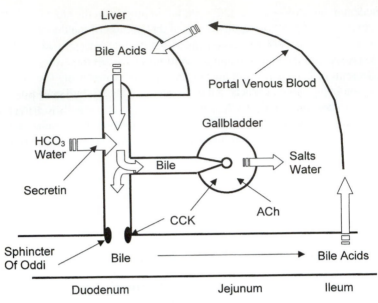

Figure 6–5
Bile acids secreted by the liver and delivered to the duodenum in bile are returned to the liver in the portal venous blood after being reabsorbed by the ileum. This is called the enterohepatic circulation.

acid, and these are called *primary bile acids.* Bacteria in the duodenum convert a small proportion of the primary bile acids to *lithocholic* and *deoxycholic* acids, which are called *secondary bile acids.*

Both primary and secondary bile acids are recycled through the *enterohepatic circulation* (see Figure 6–5). The enterohepatic circulation is a circuit followed by bile acids that includes the liver, gallbladder, small intestine, and portal venous blood. The small intestine absorbs about 95% of the secreted bile acids, which are returned to the liver in the portal vein blood. The liver effectively (100%) removes these bile acids from the blood through an Na cotransport system. Using an active transport process, the liver then returns these bile acids to the bile. In this way, bile acids cycle through the liver and intestine several times during a meal.

The gallbladder stores and concentrates the bile secreted by the liver. The liver continuously secretes bile, which accumulates in the gallbladder between meals because the opening of the bile duct into the duodenum is closed by the sphincter of Oddi. The epithelial cells of the gallbladder reabsorb Na from the bile causing Cl ions and water to follow to maintain electrical neutrality and osmotic equilibrium, respectively. In this way, bile remains isotonic even though its volume is reduced.

Regulation

- Liver continuously synthesizes and secretes the components of bile.
- Synthesis of bile acids by the liver is negatively regulated by the bile acid concentration of portal venous blood.
- Secretin increases the volume and bicarbonate concentration of bile.
- Cholecystokinin and increased vagal nerve activity increase the release of bile from the gallbladder.

The synthesis of bile acids by the liver is regulated primarily by the concentration of bile acids returning to the liver in the portal venous blood. Synthesis is reduced as the concentration of bile acid in portal blood increases. Therefore, during a meal, when the bile acid content of portal blood is high, synthesis is reduced but during the interdigestive period, when the blood content is low, synthesis is increased.

Secretin, released from the stomach in response to acid, stimulates bile duct cells to increase their secretion of water and bicarbonate ions (see Figure 6–5). *Cholecystokinin (CCK)* release from the I cells of the small intestine is increased by fat and protein in the duodenum and causes contraction of the gallbladder smooth muscle and relaxation of the sphincter of Oddi. In addition, *vagal nerve activity* to gallbladder smooth muscle increases, stimulating contraction of the gallbladder.

DIGESTION AND ABSORPTION
General Organization

- Small intestine is primary site for digestion and absorption of food.
- Surface area of small intestine is greatly increased by extensive folding and the projection of fingerlike villi covered with microvilli.
- Digestion occurs in the lumen by secreted enzymes and on surface of enterocytes by membrane-bound enzymes.
- Absorption occurs by diffusion, facilitated diffusion, active transport, endocytosis, and paracellular transport.

The small intestine is the primary organ for the digestion and absorption of food. The digestive and absorptive capacity of the small intestine so greatly exceeds demand that over 60% of the small intestine can be removed without significantly altering the absorption of carbohydrates and proteins. Only if the ileum is removed will the absorption of vitamin B_{12} and fats be impaired.

The structure of the small intestine and its cells maximizes digestion and absorption by providing a large surface area. The small intestine is extensively folded with the folds covered in fingerlike projections called *villi*. *Enterocytes*, specialized epithelial cells, cover the villi. Enterocytes further increase the surface area with hairlike projections termed *microvilli* or the *brush border*. Because of these structural features, the surface area of the small intestine is greater than that of a basketball court.

Digestion occurs in the lumen and on the surface of the enterocytes. Enzymes for luminal digestion come from secretions of the salivary glands, stomach, and pancreas with only those from the pancreas being essential. Additional enzymes are incorporated in the luminal surface of the enterocytes.

Absorption, the uptake of substances by intestinal cells, occurs through a variety of processes. The specific process depends upon the chemical nature of the substances and the physical properties of the epithelial cells. In general, absorption occurs though diffusion, facilitated diffusion, active transport, and paracellular transport.

Carbohydrate Digestion and Absorption

- Ingested carbohydrates in the form of starch are converted to glucose, galactose, or fructose by the combined action of luminal amylase and enzymes on the surface of enterocytes.
- Carbohydrate metabolites are absorbed by Na-dependent secondary active transport or facilitated diffusion across the luminal surface of enterocytes and by facilitated diffusion across the basolateral surface.

Ingested carbohydrates in the form of starch have to be reduced to individual molecules of glucose, galactose, or fructose before absorption can occur. This process begins by the action of amylase (salivary and pancreatic), which breaks the starch into short chains of sugar. These are further broken down to individual molecules of glucose, galactose, or fructose by the action of enzymes on the surface of the brush border. Amylase alone is inadequate for the digestion of carbohydrates.

Enterocytes absorb glucose and galactose through an Na-dependent secondary active transport process, while fructose is absorbed by facilitated transport (see Figure 6–6). The Na-K ion pump produces a low intracellular Na ion concentration. The diffusion of Na into the enterocyte down this gradient carries with it a molecule of glucose or galactose (secondary active transport). Once in the cell, these molecules move across the basolateral membrane by facilitated diffusion. Fructose moves across both the luminal and basolateral membranes by facilitated diffusion. As these molecules move into the intercellular spaces, they

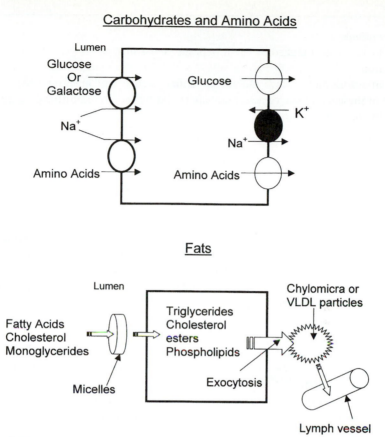

Figure 6–6

The absorption of carbohydrates and amino acids makes use of specific carrier molecules that are driven by the movement of Na ions into the cell. Fatty acids diffuse into intestinal epithelial cells from micelles and are secreted into the lymph as either chylomicra or very low density lipoprotein (VLDL) particles.

diffuse across the capillary endothelium into the blood and are carried by the portal venous blood to the liver.

Protein Digestion and Absorption

- Protein digestion begins in the stomach with the action of pepsin and is completed by proteases secreted by the pancreas, as well as by those on the surface or within the cytoplasm of enterocytes.

(continued)

> *(continued)*
> - Proteins are reduced to small peptides and amino acids prior to absorption.
> - Small peptides and individual amino acids are absorbed by Na-dependent secondary active transport and by facilitated diffusion across the basolateral surface.

Protein digestion begins in the stomach with the action of pepsin and is completed by proteases secreted by the pancreas (trypsinogen, chymotrypsinogen, procarboxypeptidase) as well as those on the surface and within the enterocytes. Pepsin is not required for protein digestion. Proteases are secreted in an inactive form. As described before, stomach acid activates pepsin. *Enterokinase*, a protease bound to the brush border of enterocytes, converts pancreatic *trypsinogen* to its active form, *trypsin.* Trypisn then converts other secreted pancreatic proteases to their active forms as well as trypsinogen to trypsin.

Proteins are degraded to short peptides consisting of 2 or 3 amino acids as well as to individual amino acids by proteases. The short peptides and amino acids are absorbed across the luminal surface of the enterocyte by an Na-dependent secondary active transport system similar to that described for carbohydrate absorption (see Figure 6–6). The transporters for carbohydrates and amino acids are distinct and transport either carbohydrates or amino acids. The uptake of short peptides utilizes carriers that are distinct from those for amino acids. Once within the enterocyte, short peptides are converted to individual amino acids and all amino acids leave the basolateral surface through a facilitated transport process. As with carbohydrates, reabsorbed amino acids diffuse from the interstitial space across the capillary endothelium and are carried to the liver by the portal venous blood.

Lipid Digestion and Absorption

- Water insolubility of lipids presents special problems for digestion and absorption, which are overcome by emulsification and formation of micelles.
- Pancreatic enzymes are primarily responsible for digesting ingested lipids to cholesterol, fatty acids, and monoglycerides.
- Enterocytes resynthesize triglycerides and phospholipids from absorbed fatty acids and monoglycerides.
- Within enterocytes, triglycerides, phospholipids, and cholesterol are packaged into chylomicra or very low density lipoproteins (VLDL) and secreted by exocytosis across the basolateral membrane.
- Chylomicra and VLDL enter the blood through lymphatic vessels draining the small intestine because they are too large to cross the capillary endothelium.

The water insolubility of ingested lipids presents a problem for digestion and absorption. Ingested lipids are composed primarily of triglycerides, phospholipids, and cholesterol esters, which are insoluble in water. Ingested lipids are first *emulsified*, that is, they are prevented from coming together in large droplets by forming complexes with amphipathic molecules. Because amphipathic molecules have both water-soluble and water-insoluble portions, they keep ingested lipids in small water-soluble droplets. Bile acids, phospholipids, monoglycerides, and proteins are important emulsifying agents in the GI tract. Emulsified lipids have a larger surface area thereby exposing more of the ingested lipids to digestive enzymes.

As the lipids are digested to fatty acids, cholesterol, and monoglycerides in the small intestine, they are complexed with bile salts to form small disclike structures called *micelles* (see Figure 6–6). Micelles are capable of diffusing through the unstirred water layer at the surface of enterocytes, which brings the digested lipids in contact with the cell surface. This contact is essential for absorption.

Pancreatic enzymes are critical for lipid digestion, but about 10% of digestion occurs in the stomach. The pancreas secretes 3 enzymes for lipid digestion: lipase, *cholesterol ester hydrolase* and *phospholipase A₂*. Pancreatic enzymes are in such excess that enzyme secretion has to be reduced by 80% before lipid digestion is reduced. Even so, the rate of stomach emptying is negatively influenced by the amount of lipid in the duodenum through the enterogastric reflex to maximize lipid digestion. All these enzymes remove fatty acids from triglycerides (lipases), from cholesterol esters (cholesterol ester hydrolase), or phospholipids (phospholipase A₂). The resulting products of free fatty acids, monoglycerides, and cholesterol are absorbed by enterocytes.

The fatty acids, monoglycerides, and cholesterol are complexed with bile salts into micelles, which bring these metabolites in close association with the luminal cell membrane of the enterocyte so that absorption can occur. Current evidence suggests that a carrier-mediated process is involved in absorption, but the nature of these processes has not been defined.

Absorbed fatty acids, cholesterol, and monoglycerides are converted back to triglycerides, cholesterol esters, and phospholipids within the enterocytes (see Figure 6–6). This conversion occurs within the *smooth endoplasmic reticulum*. From here, these resynthesized lipids move to the Golgi where they are packaged into *chylomicra* or *very low density lipoprotein (VLDL)* particles. Chylomicra contain all three lipid products while VLDL particles contain primarily triglycerides. Chylomicra and VLDL particles are secreted on the basolateral side of the enterocytes by exocytosis. They are too large to cross the capillary endothelium and so do not enter the blood directly. Instead, chylomicra and VLDL particles move across the more porous endothelium of lymph vessels, eventually entering the blood at the *thoracic duct*, the junction between the lymphatics and the blood supply. In addition to lipids, several proteins, called *apoproteins*, are associated with the chylomicron and VLDL. An important apoprotein is *Apo B*, which is required for the secretion of both chylomicra and VLDL. Apo B is absent in the autosomal recessive disease *abetalipoproteinemia*, which causes lipid accumulation in the enterocytes because secretion is prevented.

Handling of Vitamins, Ions, and Water

- Vitamins are absorbed in the small intestine either by a carrier-mediated process or by passive diffusion.
- Ion absorption occurs in the small intestine primarily by carrier-mediated processes similar to those seen in other tissues.
- Water absorption in the small and large intestines is passive and follows the absorption of osmotic particles.
- Small and large intestines can secrete ions and water.
- Diarrhea results from disturbances in water absorption.

Vitamins are important cofactors for many metabolic reactions but they are not synthesized by the body and, therefore, must be obtained from the diet. Vitamin absorption occurs in the small intestine. There are two types of vitamins, fat-soluble and water-soluble. Fat-soluble vitamins (A, D, E, and K) are absorbed in the same manner as lipids; they are incorporated into micelles, diffuse into the cells, and then leave the basolateral side incorporated in chylomicra. Water-soluble vitamins (B, C, thiamine, niacin, folate) are generally absorbed by carrier-mediated processes coupled to the movement of Na ions into the cell as described for glucose and amino acid absorption. Absorption of the water-soluble vitamin, B_{12}, requires the glycoprotein *intrinsic factor*. As described earlier, intrinsic factor is secreted by parietal cells in the stomach and is the only essential secretion of the stomach. Intrinsic factor binds vitamin B_{12}, preventing the vitamin from being digested by pancreatic enzymes and attaching it to a specific receptor on the luminal surface of enterocytes of the ileum. Through an unknown mechanism, this complex enters the cell enabling absorption.

Ions are absorbed in the small intestine primarily through carrier-mediated processes similar to those described in other tissues such as the kidney (see Figure 6–7). Na ions are absorbed across the luminal cell membrane by co-transport with sugars, amino acids, and Cl ions in exchange for H ions, as well as through Na-specific ion channels. This inward movement of Na ions depends upon a low intracellular Na ion concentration that is established by the Na-K ion pump in the basolateral cell membrane. Na ion absorption by co-transport dominates in the small intestine while absorption through channels is dominant in the distal colon. The intestinal Na ion channel is similar to that in the kidney and so when aldosterone levels are elevated in response to a fall in blood pressure, the intestinal channels will be opened and Na absorption will be increased. In addition to

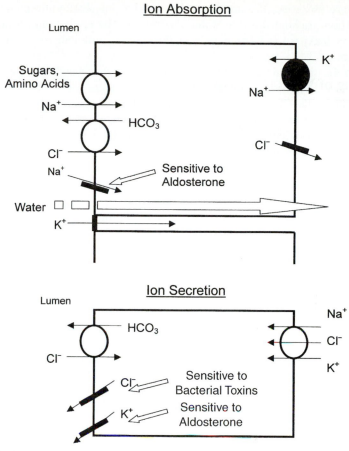

Figure 6–7
Ion absorption and secretion utilizes a variety of transport systems.

being co-transported with Na ions, Cl ions are also absorbed in exchange for intracellular bicarbonate ions in the intestine. The bicarbonate for this exchange is formed from the breakdown of carbonic acid within the enterocytes by the action of carbonic anhydrase. The same conversion was described in kidney epithelial cells. How Cl ions exit the basolateral side of the cell is unknown but is most likely by diffusion through channels. K ions are absorbed by passive diffusion through paracellular pathways. For this to occur, a concentration gradient for K must be established across the enterocytes. This occurs secondary to the absorption of water.

As in the kidney, water absorption is passive and depends upon the absorption of osmotic particles, particularly Na ions. As Na ions and other osmotic particles are absorbed, the intestinal contents become hypotonic producing a concentration gradient favoring water absorption. The epithelium of the small intestine is leaky so it takes a very small osmotic gradient to enable water absorption.

Both the small and large intestines can secrete water and ions (see Figure 6–7). As just described, bicarbonate is secreted in exchange for Cl ions. However, in some cells, Cl ions can also be secreted through specific channels. Cl ion secretion by these cells depends on a secondary active transport process. A Na-K-Cl co-transporter in the basolateral membrane of these cells brings Cl ions into the cell as Na moves down its concentration gradient. A similar tritransporter is present in the epithelial cells of the ascending thick limb of the loop of Henle. This generates a concentration gradient favoring Cl ion secretion through channels in the luminal membrane of the cell. K ions are also secreted by passive diffusion through K ion selective channels in the luminal membrane of the enterocytes. As with the Na channels, the K ion channels are opened when aldosterone levels are elevated increasing K ion secretion.

Diarrhea is caused by the inability of the intestine to absorb water. This can result from destruction of the intestinal surface so that the area available for absorption is reduced. However, since water absorption depends upon absorption of osmotic particles, diarrhea can result from the inability of enterocytes to lower the luminal osmolarity. This can occur if absorption is impaired such as with glucose-galactose malabsorption. In this case, osmotic particles, glucose and galactose, remain in the intestinal lumen and hold water. This is termed *osmotic diarrhea* and is similar to osmotic diuresis seen in the kidney. Alternatively, diarrhea occurs if intestinal secretion of osmotic particles increases. Many bacteria (*Vibrio cholerae*, some *Escherichia coli*) release toxins that open Cl channels increasing Cl ion secretion, which holds water in the intestinal lumen (see Figure 6–7). This is called *secretory diarrhea*.

ENDOCRINE PHYSIOLOGY

·

BASIC PRINCIPLES AND ORGANIZATION
Definition of the Endocrine System

- Endocrine and nervous systems coordinate complex body functions.
- Classic distinction between these two is that the endocrine system communicates to distant tissues through blood-borne chemicals while the nervous system communicates to adjacent tissue by local chemical release.
- Organs of the endocrine system include adrenal, gonads, hypothalamus, pancreas, parathyroid, pituitary, thyroid, as well as others, such as the heart, kidney, and gastrointestinal tract.

The complexity of the body requires an effective communication system for coordinating the functions of diverse organs. Both the endocrine and nervous systems provide this communication. The classic distinction between these two communication systems is that the endocrine system releases chemicals into the blood stream, which carries them to the cells of a distant target organ; in contrast, the nervous system releases chemicals into the immediate environment of the nerve ending where they act on adjacent cells within the target organ. Such a distinction is restrictive because it does not incorporate several examples where chemicals released from nerve endings act on distant organs: (1) nerves in the posterior pituitary release oxytocin and antidiuretic hormone, which act on the breast and kidneys, respectively; (2) nerves release epinephrine from the adrenal medulla, which acts on the heart, skeletal muscle, and the liver; (3) nerves of the hypothalamus secrete chemicals (releasing hormones) that act on the anterior pituitary to cause hormone release. Therefore, the definition of the endocrine system should also include such *neuroendocrine* systems.

The organs that comprise the endocrine system should also be expanded to include organs that are not part of the classical list. The heart, kidney, and gastrointestinal tract are examples of nonclassic endocrine organs. As was described in previous chapters, the heart is known to secrete the atrial natriuretic hormone, the kidney secretes erythropoietin and renin, while the GI tract secretes gastrin, secretin, and cholecystokinin (CCK). So these organs should also be considered as part of the endocrine system. In this chapter the classic endocrine organs will be discussed: adrenal, gonads, hypothalamus, pancreas, parathyroid, pituitary, and thyroid. Table 7–1 lists these organs, the hormones released, and their primary tissue effect.

TABLE 7–1 ENDOCRINE GLANDS, HORMONES SECRETED, AND TISSUE EFFECT		
ENDOCRINE GLAND	**HORMONES SECRETED**	**TISSUE EFFECT**
Hypothalamus	Corticotropin-releasing hormone (CRH)	Stimulates ACTH secretion
	Dopamine	Inhibits prolactin secretion
	Gonadotropin-releasing hormone (GnRH)	Stimulates LH and FSH secretion
	Growth-hormone releasing hormone (GHRH)	Stimulates GH secretion
	Somatostatin	Inhibits GH secretion
	Thyrotropin-releasing hormone (TRH)	Stimulates TSH and prolactin secretion
Anterior pituitary	Adrenocorticotropic hormone (ACTH)	Stimulates synthesis/secretion of cortisol, androgens, aldosterone
	Follicle-stimulating hormone (FSH)	Stimulates sperm maturation; development of ovarian follicles
	Growth hormone (GH)	Stimulates protein synthesis and growth
	Luteinizing hormone (LH)	Stimulates testosterone, estrogen, progesterone synthesis; stimulates ovulation
	Melanocyte-stimulating hormone (MSH)	Stimulates melanin synthesis
	Prolactin	Stimulates milk production
	Thyroid-stimulating hormone (TSH)	Stimulates thyroid hormone synthesis/secretion

(*continued*)

ENDOCRINE GLAND	HORMONES SECRETED	TISSUE EFFECT

TABLE 7–1   ENDOCRINE GLANDS, HORMONES SECRETED, AND TISSUE EFFECT (*continued*)

ENDOCRINE GLAND	HORMONES SECRETED	TISSUE EFFECT
Posterior pituitary	Oxytocin	Stimulates milk ejection and uterine contraction
	Antidiuretic hormone (ADH)	Stimulates renal water reabsorption
Thyroid	Triiodothyronine (T_3) and thyroxine (T_4)	Stimulates growth, oxygen consumption, heat production, metabolism, nervous system development
	Calcitonin	Decreases blood Ca concentration
Parathyroid	Parathyroid hormone (PTH)	Increases blood Ca concentration
Adrenal cortex	Cortisol	Increases glucose synthesis; mediates "stress" response
	Aldosterone	Increases renal reabsorption of Na^+, secretion of K^+ and H^+
	Androgens	Similar to testosterone but weaker
Adrenal medulla	Epinephrine	Stimulates fat and carbohydrate metabolism
Pancreas	Insulin	Decreases blood glucose levels; anabolic effects on lipid and protein metabolism
	Glucagon	Increases blood glucose levels
Testes	Testosterone	Stimulates spermatogenesis and secondary sex characteristics
Ovaries	Estradiol	Stimulates growth/development of female reproductive system and breasts, follicular phase of menstrual cycle, prolactin secretion, and maintains pregnancy
	Progesterone	Luteal phase of menstrual cycle and maintains pregnancy
Corpus luteum	Estradiol and progesterone	See above
Placenta	Human chorionic gonadotropin (hCG)	Stimulates estrogen/progesterone synthesis by corpus luteum
	Human placental lactogen (hPL)	Acts like GH and prolactin during pregnancy
	Estriol	Acts like estradiol
	Progesterone	See above

This table lists the major endocrine organs, the hormones each organ secretes, and the major tissue effect of the hormone.

Chemical Nature of Hormones

- Classic definition of a hormone is a chemical produced by an organ in a small amount that is released into the blood stream to act on cells in a distant tissue.
- This definition needs to be expanded to include chemicals that have paracrine and autocrine functions.
- Hormones are divided into four groups based on chemical structure: amines, peptides, proteins, steroids.

The original definition of a hormone is a chemical produced in small amounts, released into the blood stream, and carried to a distant site where it acts on the cells of an organ. However, we have come to learn that hormones represent a larger group of chemicals that can also have effects closer to their site of secretion. Hormones now include chemicals that act on neighboring cells in a *paracrine* function or even on the cells that secreted them in an *autocrine* function.

Hormones can be divided into four groups based on chemical structure. The members of each group are listed in Table 7–2. The *amine hormones* are derivatives of the amino acid tyrosine. *Peptide hormones* (less than 20 amino acids) and small *protein hormones* (greater than 20 amino acids) are composed of sequences of amino acids. *Steroid hormones* are derivatives of cholesterol.

Mechanism of Hormone Action

- Hormones act through specific receptors that define tissue selectivity and response.
- Receptors for amine, protein, and peptide hormones are located on the cell membrane, while those for steroid and thyroid hormones are within the cell.
- Membrane receptors are of four types based on their signaling mechanism: G protein, tyrosine kinase, guanylyl cyclase, cytokine family.
- Steroid and thyroid hormones act through nuclear receptors that stimulate gene expression.
- Membrane-receptor mediated hormones elicit rapid cellular responses; nuclear-receptor mediated hormones elicit slow, long lasting cellular responses.

For a hormone to produce a cellular response, the cell must possess a receptor for that hormone. Tissue sensitivity to a hormone is therefore dependent on the type of receptor(s) the tissue possesses.

TABLE 7–2 MAJOR HORMONES GROUPED BY CHEMICAL STRUCTURE			
AMINES	**PEPTIDES**	**PROTEINS**	**STEROIDS**
Dopamine	Antidiuretic hormone	Adrenocorticotropic	Aldosterone
Epinephrine	(ADH)	hormone (ACTH)	Cortisol
Thyroxine	Gonadotropin-	Calcitonin	Estradiol
(T_4)	releasing hormone	Human chorionic go-	Estriol
Triiodothy-	(GnRH)	nadotropin (hCG)	Progesterone
ronine (T_3)	Melanocyte-	Human placental	Testosterone
	stimulating	lactogen (hPL)	1,25-vitamin D
	hormone (MSH)	Corticotropin-releasing	
	Oxytocin	hormone (CRH)	
	Thyrotropin-releasing	Glucagon	
	hormone (TRH)	Growth hormone (GH)	
	Somatostatin	Growth hormone-	
		releasing hormone	
		(GHRH)	
		Follicle-stimulating	
		hormone (FSH)	
		Insulin	
		Insulin-like growth	
		factor (IGF-1)	
		Luteinizing hormone	
		(LH)	
		Parathyroid hormone	
		(PTH)	
		Prolactin	
		Thyroid-stimulating	
		hormone (TSH)	

This table groups the major hormones according to their chemical composition.

The different classes of hormones operate through different types of receptors. For the amines (thyroid hormones are an exception), protein, and peptide hormones the receptors reside on the cell surface, while for the steroid and thyroid hormones the receptors are intracellular.

Membrane receptors consist of three components: (1) an extracellular domain that binds the hormone; (2) a transmembrane domain that anchors it in the membrane; and (3) an intracellular domain that couples the receptor to an intracellular signaling system. For the G-protein coupled receptors (described below), the transmembrane domain loops back and forth through the membrane 7 times while for others it passes through only once. When the hormone stimulates the receptor, an intracellular signaling system is activated that initiates a cascade of cellular events culminating in the hormone response.

Membrane receptors are grouped into four types based on their intracellular signaling mechanisms. Membrane receptor types are listed in Table 7–3 along with the hormones that activate them. *G-protein linked receptors* have the characteristic of being linked to an intracellular class of proteins called *G proteins*. G proteins are a cluster of three proteins that, when activated by hormone binding to the extracellular domain of the receptor, cause stimulation of one of two enzymes, *adenylyl cyclase* or *phospholipase C*. Activation of adenylyl cyclase leads to the formation of *cyclic adenosine monophosphate (cyclic AMP)*, and activation of phospholipase C leads to the formation of *inositol trisphosphate (IP$_3$)* or *diacylglyercerol (DAG)*, or activation of *protein kinase C (PKC)*. These second messenger molecules initiate a cascade of events culminating in the hormone response.

The *tyrosine kinase receptors* are distinguished by having an intracellular domain that phosphorylates proteins on specific tyrosine molecules. These tyrosine-phosphorylated proteins act as second messengers to initiate a cascade of events leading to hormone response.

The *guanylyl cyclase receptors* have the enzyme *guanylyl cyclase* as a portion of their intracellular domain. Binding of hormone to the extracellular

TABLE 7–3   HORMONES SIGNALING THROUGH MEMBRANE RECEPTORS

G-Protein Receptors Linked to:		Tyrosine Kinase Receptors	Guanylyl Cyclase Receptors	Cytokine Receptor Family
Adenylyl Cyclase	**Phospholipase C**			
ACTH, calcitonin, CRH, dopamine, epinephrine, FSH, glucagon, hCG, LH, MSH, PTH, somatostatin, TSH	ADH, GHRH, GnRH, oxytocin, TRH	Insulin, insulin-like growth factor-1 (IGF-1)	ANP	GH, prolactin

This table groups the major hormones according to their signaling mechanisms.

domain leads to activation of guanylyl cyclase and the formation of *cyclic guanosine monophosphate (cyclic GMP)*. This second messenger initiates the hormone response.

The final group of membrane receptors belongs to a large class of receptors called the *cytokine receptor family*. This family is distinguished by the fact that receptor activation indirectly leads to intracellular protein tyrosine phosphorylation. Hormone binding to the extracellular receptor domain enables the intracellular domain to bind soluble tyrosine kinases called *Janus kinases* (or *JAK kinases*). Binding activates the JAK kinases, which phosphorylate intracellular proteins and produce the hormone response.

Steroid and thyroid hormones (primarily T_3) signal through intracellular receptors, which act solely to initiate gene expression. Both hormone types diffuse through the cell membrane to act on their intracellular receptors. The receptors are protein molecules that bind to specific DNA sequences known as *hormone response elements (HRE)*. The hormone-receptor complex activates the HRE, initiating DNA transcription leading to protein synthesis.

Because of the nature of the signaling mechanisms, the tissue response to membrane-receptor mediated hormones is more rapid (minutes) than is the response of nuclear-receptor mediated hormones (hours). The increase in protein synthesis elicited by nuclear-mediated receptors takes hours to occur but is long lasting since termination of the response requires protein degradation.

Synthesis and Release of Hormones

> • Peptide and protein hormones are synthesized from amino acids as prohormones or preprohormones, which are subsequently modified and stored in vesicles until secreted by exocytosis.
> • Amine and steroid hormones are synthesized from precursor molecules (tyrosine, cholesterol) present in the blood.
> • Thyroid and steroid hormones are not stored in secretory vesicles, but the amine hormone epinephrine is.

Peptide and protein hormones are synthesized from amino acids in the rough endoplasmic reticulum (rough ER) of the cell as either a *prohormone* or a *preprohormone*. Both of these initial forms of a hormone molecule contain an amino acid sequence that makes them fat-soluble so they can move across the membrane of the rough ER into the Golgi apparatus. Preprohormones have additional internal cleavage sites that are removed to produce hormones of different biological action. Once in the Golgi apparatus, these molecules are enzymatically converted to the active form of the hormone and stored in vesicles for secretion by exocytosis.

Amine and steroid hormones are synthesized from the precursor molecules tyrosine and cholesterol, respectively. In general, amine and steroid hormones are synthesized on demand and are not stored in vesicles in the active form. An exception is the amine hormone, epinephrine, which is stored in vesicles and secreted by exocytosis.

Control of Hormone Release

> • Most hormones are released in a pulsatile manner with a frequency that varies from minutes to months and is characteristic of the hormone.
> • Hormone release is influenced in part by positive and negative feedback mechanisms.

Most hormones are released in a pulsatile manner that varies in frequency from minutes to months. This pulsatile release is the consequence of the intrinsic secretory properties of the endocrine cells combined with complex feedback mechanisms.

Both negative and positive feedback mechanisms influence hormone release with negative feedback being the most common. In negative feedback some aspect of hormone action inhibits further release of hormone. The simplest example is an inhibitory effect by the hormone itself. As the plasma concentration of the hormone rises, this increasing concentration begins to inhibit its further release, usually by inhibiting synthesis and secretion of the trophic hormone that regulates it. However, negative feedback can be very complex involving a multitude of hormones from a variety of organs acting at multiple levels of higher control. Positive feedback systems enhance further hormone release and achieve a maximum level of hormone release that is limited by the secretory capacity of the tissue.

Hormone Transport in the Blood

> • Amine, peptide, and small protein hormones circulate in a free form in blood because they are water soluble.
> • Steroid and thyroid hormones are carried in the blood bound to proteins because they are water insoluble.
> • Only the free form of the hormone can stimulate tissue receptors.
> • Most hormones are removed from the blood by the liver and kidney shortly after being secreted even though their tissue effect continues.

Amine (except thyroid hormone), peptide, and small protein hormones are in a free form in the blood because they are water-soluble. In contrast, steroid and thyroid hormones are bound to proteins in the blood because they are insoluble in water. Some carrier proteins are hormone specific while others, such as albumin, bind a variety of hormones. Protein binding reduces hormone loss through the kidney since the protein-hormone complex cannot be filtered. Protein-bound hormones must dissociate from the carrier protein before they can induce a cellular response, because only free hormones can cross the capillary endothelium and stimulate tissue receptors.

Shortly after being secreted, hormones are removed from the blood primarily by the liver and kidneys. The rate at which the amount of hormone in blood decreases is called its *half-life*. This is the time it takes the concentration of the hormone to fall to one half of its previous level. Half-lives vary from minutes for the amine hormones to hours for steroid and thyroid hormones. The blood hormone concentration decreases at a faster rate than does the hormone response. This is because hormones initiate a cascade of events within the cell that once initiated do not require the continuous presence of the hormone.

HYPOTHALAMUS AND THE PITUITARY GLAND
General Organization

- Pituitary gland and hypothalamus function in a coordinated manner to integrate many endocrine glands.
- Pituitary gland is located just below the hypothalamus at the base of the brain to which it is connected by a short stalk.
- Pituitary is divided into anterior and posterior portions.
- Secretion of anterior pituitary hormones is under the control of hypothalamic releasing hormones.
- Posterior pituitary hormones are synthesized in hypothalamic nerves that end in the posterior pituitary where hormone is released into the blood.

The action of many endocrine glands is coordinated through the combined action of the pituitary gland and hypothalamus. The pituitary gland, divided into anterior and posterior portions, is located below and connected to the hypothalamus by a short stalk called the *infundibulum*.

Hormone secretion of the anterior pituitary is under control of releasing hormones from the hypothalamus. Nerves of the hypothalamus synthesize and secrete *releasing hormones* into the blood supply of the anterior pituitary. Hypothalamic releasing hormones stimulate secretion of specific anterior pituitary hormones.

In contrast, secretions of the posterior pituitary are from nerve endings that originate in the hypothalamus. Axons of nerve cell bodies in the hypothalamus extend through the infundibulum into the posterior pituitary where they end and release their hormones into the venous blood of the posterior pituitary. From there they circulate throughout the body.

Hypothalamic Hormones Influence Anterior Pituitary Hormone Secretion

> Six hormones are released from the hypothalamus that control the release of anterior pituitary hormones: TRH, dopamine, GnRH, CRH, GHRH, somatostatin.

Clusters of nerve cells within the hypothalamus produce one of six different hormones (releasing hormones) that alter the secretion of specific hormone-producing cells *(trophic cells)* of the anterior pituitary (see Figure 7–1).

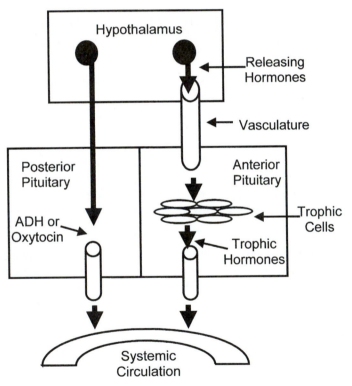

Figure 7–1
The hypothalamus regulates secretions from both the anterior and posterior pituitary. In the anterior pituitary, this is accomplished through the release of hypothalamic-releasing factors. In the posterior pituitary, the secretions are released from nerves that originate in the hypothalamus.

(1) *Thyrotropin-releasing hormone (TRH)* acts on the thyrotrophs and lactotrophs stimulating TSH and prolactin secretion, respectively. (2) *Dopamine* inhibits lactotroph secretion of prolactin. (3) *Gonadotropin hormone-releasing hormone (GnRH)* stimulates FSH and LH secretion from the gonadotrophs. (4) *Corticotropin-releasing hormone (CRH)* stimulates corticotroph secretion of ACTH. (5) *Growth hormone-releasing hormone (GHRH)* and (6) *somatostatin* both act on anterior pituitary somatotrophs with GHRH stimulating and somatostatin inhibiting GH secretion.

Anterior Pituitary Hormones

- Seven hormones are secreted by groups of anterior pituitary cells: TSH, FSH, LH, ACTH, MSH, GH, prolactin.
- Trophic action is the primary effect of anterior pituitary hormones.
- Anterior pituitary hormones can be organized into three groups based on chemical and functional similarities: TSH, FSH, LH; ACTH and MSH; GH and prolactin.
- GH is the main regulator of postnatal growth and development, and prolactin is the major hormone responsible for milk production.

The anterior pituitary secretes seven hormones that are peptides or small proteins (see Table 7–2). Anterior pituitary hormones are *trophic hormones*, that is, their effect is to change the morphology and secretory action of other endocrine glands or tissues. Specific anterior pituitary cells secrete these hormones, and these cell groups are called: *thyrotrophs* (TSH); *gonadotrophs* (FSH and LH); *corticotrophs* (ACTH, MSH); *somatotrophs* (GH); and *lactotrophs* (prolactin). The hormones they secrete can be organized into three groups based on chemical and functional similarities: (1) FSH, LH, and TSH; (2) ACTH and MSH; (3) GH and prolactin.

FSH, LH, and TSH are each composed of two amino acid chains that are chemically linked together. One amino acid chain (α-chain) is identical in all three hormones while the other chain (β-chain) varies, giving each hormone its specific physiology action. FSH and LH act on the gonads of both females and males to stimulate their development and hormone secretion. TSH maintains the size of thyroid cells and stimulates the secretion of both thyroid hormones. More details on the action of these hormones are provided in the sections on reproduction and the thyroid gland.

ACTH and MSH are derived from a single precursor molecule, *pro-opiomelanocortin (POMC)*, that is enzymatically modified within the corticotroph cells to yield the individual hormones. In humans little if any MSH is produced as a specific hormone, however, ACTH contains a short form of MSH in its amino acid sequence. A consequence of this is that when ACTH levels are very high *(Addison's disease)*, they will have MSH activity causing the skin to darken because of melanocyte simulation. Recent evidence suggests that alpha-MSH and other POMC products may be involved in hypothalamic-neural circuits that regulate appetite and energy balance. ACTH maintains the size of cells in the adrenal cortex and stimulates the secretion of cortisol from the cortex. Additional information about ACTH is included in the section on the adrenal gland.

GH and prolactin are both straight amino acid chains that are about 75% identical. Even though GH and prolactin are not strictly trophic hormones since they do not act on other endocrine organs, GH is essential for normal body growth and prolactin for milk synthesis by mammary glands.

GH is the main regulator of postnatal growth and development. Blood levels are cyclical, with surges in secretion occurring at night during sleep. These surges are under the reciprocal control of GHRH (stimulatory) and somatostatin (inhibitory) release from the hypothalamus, which in turn is regulated by higher brain centers as well as by blood levels of GHRH and GH. GHRH has a negative feedback effect limiting its own secretion from the hypothalamus. GH limits its own secretion by stimulating somatostatin released from the hypothalamus (see Figure 7–2). GH has effects on metabolism that result from the direct action of GH on target tissue and effects on growth through GH release of *insulin-like growth factor 1 (IGF-1)* primarily from the liver. GH's metabolic effects include decreased tissue glucose uptake with a consequential increase in blood glucose levels; increased fat metabolism by adipose tissue; and increased tissue amino acid uptake. These metabolic effects lead to an increase in lean body mass and to an elevation in blood insulin levels. IGF-1 stimulates cell division in many tissues especially bone. Its effect on bone produces linear growth. In addition, IGF-1 stimulates protein synthesis facilitated by the increased amino acid uptake produced by GH. Given these normal effects, it follows that GH deficiency

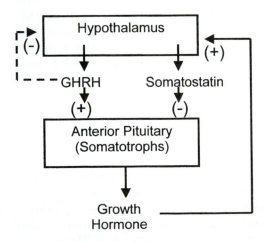

Figure 7–2
The control of growth hormone release occurs at both the hypothalamic and anterior pituitary levels.

during early childhood results in a child with a short stature and excess body fat, while overproduction *(acromegaly)* results in excess organ and linear growth.

Prolactin is the major hormone responsible for milk production *(lactogenesis)* and is involved in breast development. Prolactin secretion is reciprocally controlled through the stimulatory actions of TRH (and other yet to be identified hormones) and the inhibitory effect of dopamine. In the nonlactating person, the effect of dopamine dominates so blood levels of prolactin are low. At puberty in the female, prolactin enhances the ability of the elevated levels of estrogen and progesterone to stimulate breast development. During pregnancy, prolactin secretion increases, and together with estrogen and progesterone enhance the development of milk-producing cells in the breast. Despite the high prolactin levels, milk production does not occur because the high levels of estrogen and progesterone act on the mammary gland to block the lactogenic effect of prolactin. At birth, the mother's blood levels of prolactin, estrogen, and progesterone fall. The act of suckling stimulates TRH (or some other factor) and inhibits dopamine release producing a surge of prolactin secretion, which stimulates milk production.

Posterior Pituitary

> Posterior pituitary secretes two hormones, oxytocin and antidiuretic hormone, that are synthesized by nerves in the paraventricular and supraoptic nuclei of the hypothalamus.

In the hypothalamus two clusters of nerve cells, *paraventricular* and *supraoptic nuclei*, synthesize *oxytocin* and *antidiuretic hormone (ADH)* (see Figure 7–1). Both hormones are synthesized as preprohormones, packaged in vesicles where they are enzymatically converted to prohormones. Axons from these nuclei extend into the posterior pituitary and end adjacent to the gland's blood supply. The vesicles containing the prohormones migrate down the axons to the nerve endings in the posterior pituitary where the active hormone is formed. Upon stimulation the vesicles fuse with the axon membrane and release their contents into the blood stream.

Oxytocin causes milk ejection in response to suckling by stimulating contraction of myoepithelial cells lining the ducts leading to the nipples. Sensory receptors in the nipples signal the brain and hypothalamus causing activation of nerve cells of the paraventricular nucleus and oxytocin release. In addition, oxytocin stimulates uterine contraction but its role in parturition is unclear. ADH increases water reabsorption by increasing the water permeability of the collecting duct of the kidney. Further discussion of its mechanism of action and the control of its release can be found in chapter 4, Renal Physiology.

THYROID GLAND
General Organization

> - Thyroid gland consists of two lobes, one on either side of the trachea just below the cricoid cartilage.
> - Lobes are composed of spherical follicles formed by a single layer of epithelial cells that surround a lumen filled with a gel-like substance called colloid composed primarily of thyroglobulin, the precursor of thyroid hormones.

The thyroid gland consists of two lobes, one on either side of the trachea just below the cricoid cartilage. Each lobe consists of spherical follicles with capillaries between each follicle. The walls of the follicle are composed of a single layer of epithelial cells. The lumen of the sphere is filled with a substance called *colloid*, which is composed primarily of *thyroglobulin*, the precursor of the thyroid hormones. The epithelial cells synthesize and secrete thyroglobulin.

Synthesis of Thyroid Hormone

> - Synthesis includes steps that occur within the epithelial cells and colloid of the thyroid gland as well as at the target tissue.
> - Iodine uptake and thyroglobulin synthesis occur within epithelial cells.
> - Iodination of thyroglobulin and synthesis of T_3 and T_4 occur within the colloid.
> - T_3, most active form of the hormone, is produced from T_4 at the target tissue.

The synthesis of T_3, the most active form of the hormone, is a complex process involving many sites (see Figure 7–3). It begins with the uptake of iodide ions (I^-) from the blood by epithelial cells of the follicle via an active transport system that co-transports Na^+ ions into the cell. Inside the cell, iodide ions are oxidized to molecules of iodine (I_2) by *thyroid peroxidase*. Thyroglobulin, synthesized within the epithelial cells, is a large protein composed of many tyrosine molecules. Thyroglobulin and I_2 are both secreted into the lumen of the follicle where I_2 is chemically combined with some of the tyrosines of thyroglobulin to form *monoiodotyrosine (MIT)* and *diiodotyrosine (DIT)*. Some of MIT and DIT combine to form T_3 and some DIT combines to form T_4. Ten times more T_4 is formed than T_3 because the combination of two DIT molecules is much faster.

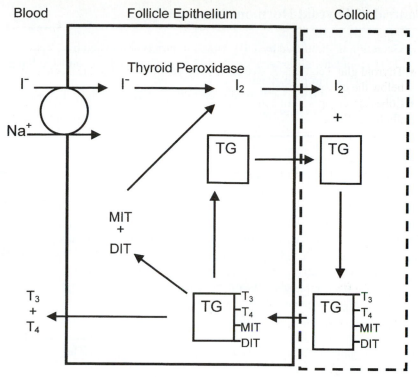

Figure 7–3
Thyroid hormone synthesis and secretion involves processes that occur within follicular epithelial cells and in colloid.

All these molecules remain part of the thyroglobulin and form the colloid in the lumen of the follicle.

Stimulation of hormone secretion by TSH causes the epithelial cells to engulf small globs of colloid and move them into the cell by endocytosis. Within the epithelial cell, MIT, DIT, T_3, and T_4 are enzymatically removed from the thyroglobulin. T_3 and T_4 are secreted into the blood while MIT and DIT are broken down to I^- and tyrosine molecules for reuse by the epithelial cell.

Most of the secreted T_3 and T_4 are carried in the blood bound to *thyroxine-binding globulin (TBG)*. T_3 is more biologically active than T_4, but since T_4 synthesis occurs more rapidly, more T_4 than T_3 is secreted. Target tissues contain an enzyme, *5'-iodinase* that converts T_4 to T_3.

Control of Thyroid Hormone Secretion

- Secretion is stimulated by TSH, which in turn is stimulated by TRH.
- TSH stimulates all aspects of thyroid hormone synthesis and secretion and also has a trophic effect.
- Elevated blood levels of T_3 feed back to the anterior pituitary thyrotrophs and reduce TSH secretion.

Secretion of thyroid hormone (T_3 and T_4) is stimulated by the TSH–TRH axis. TRH is released from the hypothalamus in response to stimuli from the central nervous system. TRH acts on the anterior pituitary thyrotrophs stimulating TSH release. TSH acts on the thyroid gland stimulating every aspect of thyroid hormone synthesis and secretion. TSH increases iodide uptake by follicular cells, iodination of thyroglobulin, formation of MIT and DIT, and endocytosis of colloid. These actions are mediated through G-protein coupled membrane TSH receptors on the thyroid gland that stimulate the formation of cyclic AMP and a cascade of protein phosphorylation steps. With sustained TSH release, a trophic effect occurs causing thyroid gland enlargement.

T_3 controls its own release through a negative feedback effect on the pituitary thyrotrophs (see Figure 7–4). Increasing blood levels of free T_3 act on pituitary thyrotrophs to decrease their number of TRH receptors. This makes TRH

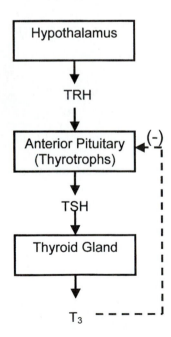

Figure 7–4
Thyroid hormone (T_3) limits its own secretion by inhibiting TSH release from thyrotroph cells of the anterior pituitary.

less effective, decreasing the amount of TSH released and therefore, the amount of thyroid hormone secreted. The net effect of this feedback process is to produce a relatively constant blood level of thyroid hormones.

Action of Thyroid Hormones

- Because T_3 acts by inducing DNA transcription, its effects on tissue are the result of protein synthesis, primarily the synthesis of enzymes.
- Thyroid hormones are required for normal growth throughout life.
- Thyroid hormones affect basal metabolic rate, metabolism, the cardio-vascular system, and the nervous system.
- Symptoms of thyroid hormone excess or deficiency can be predicted from their normal effect.

Most of the tissue effects of thyroid hormones can be attributed to the fact that their mode of action is to stimulate protein synthesis, primarily the synthesis of enzymes. Synthesis and secretion of thyroid hormones begin early in gestation and continue throughout life. Normal growth will not occur in the absence of thyroid hormones even with the presence of adequate growth hormone. Thyroid hormones stimulate the synthesis and activity of many enzymes particularly the Na-K-ATPase involved in ion transport. To support the activity of this enzyme the cell must synthesize adequate ATP, which raises the cellular oxygen consumption and heat production. In this way, thyroid hormone levels affect basal metabolic rate.

Thyroid hormones also stimulate the synthesis of many metabolic enzymes that are involved in providing substrates for ATP synthesis. So enzymes needed for glucose synthesis (gluconeogenesis) and fat and protein breakdown are increased, resulting in sustained blood glucose levels and decreased muscle mass. To deliver these substrates to the tissue requires increased cardiac output. Thyroid hormone increases heart rate and ventricular contractility by stimulating the synthesis of myosin, sarcoplasmic reticulum Ca-ATPase, and adrenergic receptors. Finally, thyroid hormones are essential for the development and normal maturation of both the central and peripheral nervous systems. The mechanisms for these effects are not fully understood.

Symptoms of excess or deficient thyroid hormone levels are predictable from their normal effects. The most common cause of excess thyroid hormone production *(hyperthyroidism)* is an autoimmune disease in which a normally produced antibody to TSH receptors, *thyroid-stimulating immunoglobulin*, is produced in excess causing intense stimulation of the thyroid gland. This is known as *Graves' disease.* Symptoms include weight loss accompanied by increased appetite, increased oxygen consumption, rapid heart and breathing rates, and nervousness. The most common cause of thyroid hormone deficiency is autoimmune destruction of the thyroid gland *(thyroiditis)*. Symptoms include weight loss, decreased basal metabolic rate, decreased heart rate, and decreased physical and mental activity. If hypothyroidism occurs early in development, irreversible retardation of growth and mental ability *(cretinism)* occurs.

ADRENAL GLAND
General Organization

> * The adrenal gland, located above each kidney, is divided into an outer cortex and an inner medulla.
> * The adrenal cortex secretes three classes of steroid hormones—mineralocorticoids, glucocorticoids and androgens—each from a different cell layer.
> * The adrenal medulla secretes the catecholamines, epinephrine, and norepinephrine.

The adrenal gland is divided into an outer cortex and an inner medulla. The cortex is divided into three layers (see Figure 7–5): (1) *zona glomerulosa* (outer layer), which secretes the *mineralocorticosteroid, aldosterone*; (2) *zona fasciculata*, which secretes the *glucocorticoid, cortisol*; and (3) *zona reticularis* (inner layer), which secretes the *androgens, dehydroepinandrosterone* and *androstenedione*.

The adrenal medulla secretes the catecholamines, epinephrine, and norepinephrine with more epinephrine than norepinephrine being released.

Adrenal Cortex

Hormone Synthesis

> * Hormones of the cortex are all derived from cholesterol.
> * Each cortical layer possesses unique enzymes that permit the synthesis of layer-specific hormones from the common precursor, pregnenolone.

All adrenocortical hormones are synthesized from cholesterol, which is obtained primarily from the blood. The enzymes for adrenal steroid hormone synthesis belong to a large family of enzymes called *P450 oxidases*. The initial and rate limiting step common to the synthesis of all adrenocortical hormones is the formation of *pregnenolone* through the action of *cholesterol desmolase (P450scc)*. The activity of this enzyme is under the control of ACTH. Each cell layer has unique enzymes that enable the layer to synthesize its unique hormone from pregnenolone (see Figure 7–5).

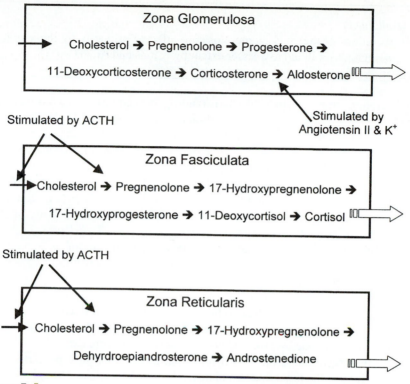

Figure 7–5
Each zone of the adrenal cortex utilizes different enzymes to synthesize specific hormones from cholesterol. ACTH primarily stimulates secretions from the zona fasciculata and reticularis while angiotensin II and K ions stimulate secretion from the zona glomerulosa.

Control of Hormone Secretion

- Secretions of the zona fasciculata and reticularis are under the sole control of the CRH–ACTH axis.
- Cortisol secretion from the zona fasciculata is pulsatile with a diurnal rhythm driven by activity within the brain.
- Stress stimulates the hypothalamus–pituitary–adrenal axis to increase cortisol secretion.
- Cortisol secretion is limited by a negative feedback system at the level of both the hypothalamus and anterior pituitary.

(continued)

(*continued*)
* Secretions of the zona glomerulosa are affected primarily by the action of angiotensin II and to a lesser extent by K ions and ACTH.

The secretions from the zona reticularis (androgens) and fasciculata (cortisol) are both controlled by the hypothalamic–pituitary axis through CRH–ACTH. CRH, released from the hypothalamus, stimulates ACTH release from the anterior pituitary through a G protein coupled membrane receptor. Activation of the CRH receptor leads to phosphorylation of proteins that increase ACTH secretion and stimulation of the gene responsible for POMC synthesis, the precursor of ACTH. In both the zona reticularis and fasciculata, ACTH acts through G protein coupled membrane receptors to increase cholesterol uptake and the activity of cholesterol desmolase (P450scc) raising the levels of pregnenolone. Within each cell layer, different P450 enzymes act upon pregnenolone or one of its byproducts (see Figure 7–5). The zona reticularis contains P450c17, which has two actions on pregnenolone. First it adds an OH group (*17α-hydroxylase* activity) and then it removes a carbon side chain (*17,20-lyase* activity) resulting in the formation of the androgen dehydroepinandrosterone. This is converted to a second androgen, androstenedione. The zona fasciculata contains P450c11 (*11β-hydroxylase*), which acts on a pregnenolone by-product, 11-deoxycortisol, to form cortisol.

Cortisol secretion is pulsatile with a diurnal variation driven by rhythmic neural activity in the brain that stimulates pulsatile CRH release. Blood levels of cortisol are highest immediately before waking and shortly thereafter. Stress and other stimuli override this pattern by directly increasing CRH–ACTH–cortisol secretion. Under such conditions, blood levels of cortisol feed back and reduce further secretion by inhibiting CRH release, CRH action on anterior pituitary corticotrophs, and if sustained, the synthesis of POMC (see Figure 7–6).

Aldosterone secretion by the zona glomerulosa is stimulated primarily by angiotensin II and to a lesser extent by K ions and the CRH–ACTH axis. ACTH stimulates pregnenolone synthesis as in other adrenocortical layers, which can lead to increased aldosterone synthesis by providing increased levels of hormone precursor. However, the zona glomerulosa contains a unique enzyme, *aldosterone synthase* (a form of P450c11), which is directly activated by angiotensin II and to a lesser extent by elevated K ions (see Figure 7–5). This enzyme converts corticosterone to aldosterone. Both angiotensin II and elevated K ions activate aldosterone synthase by initiating a Ca-dependent protein phosphorylation cascade. Angiotensin II elevates Ca through a G protein coupled receptor while elevated extracellular K depolarizes the cells causing Ca influx. It makes sense that angiotensin II stimulates aldosterone secretion because aldosterone increases renal salt reabsorption, which would restore a reduced extracellular volume, one

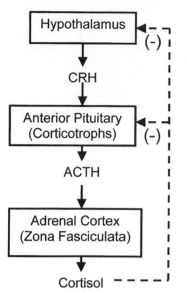

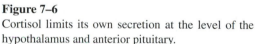

Figure 7–6
Cortisol limits its own secretion at the level of the hypothalamus and anterior pituitary.

of the stimuli for angiotensin II formation. Also, since aldosterone stimulates renal K ion secretion, an elevated aldosterone level induced by high blood K would help normalize blood K concentration. Refer to chapter 4, Renal Physiology, to review extracellular volume control through the renin-angiotensin II-aldosterone system and the mechanism by which aldosterone stimulates renal K ion secretion.

Glucocorticoid Action

> • Glucocorticoids (cortisol) are essential for life.
> • Glucocorticoids are catabolic and diabetogenic, reduce inflammation, suppress immune responses, and support vascular response to catecholamines.

We cannot survive without glucocorticoid secretion from the adrenal cortex. The overall metabolic effect of cortisol is to increase blood glucose levels, which is accomplished by increasing glucose synthesis and reducing glucose utilization. Therefore, cortisol plays an important role during fasting and starvation. Cortisol, glucagon, growth hormone, and epinephrine all act to prevent a fall in blood glucose level that is, *hypoglycemia*.

Cortisol secretion is controlled in several ways. As indicated above, cortisol secretion exhibits a daily pattern of basal secretion in which secretion increases upon waking. However, secretion is increased in response to hypoglycemia, stress, and trauma. This increase in secretion is mediated primarily through the hypothalamus—anterior pituitary axis, that is, through CRH–ACTH.

Cortisol (see Figure 7–7) stimulates the breakdown of protein in muscle and fat in adipose tissue, thereby making amino acids and glycerol available for glucose synthesis in the liver. In addition, cortisol reduces glucose utilization by skeletal muscle and fat cells. This occurs by a direct action of the hormone on these cells and by inhibiting insulin stimulation of glucose uptake by fat cells. This spares blood glucose for the central nervous system, an obligatory glucose user. Other tissues shift to fatty acid metabolism for their energy needs since their uptake of glucose has been reduced by cortisol. The primary mechanism of action for these metabolic effects is through gene induction with subsequent synthesis of specific proteins that mediate the effects. In some cases these proteins may be stimulatory while in others they may be inhibitory.

Cortisol also interferes with the body's inflammatory response by reducing the synthesis of substances that mediate the inflammatory response such as prostaglandins, leukotrienes, interleukin-2, histamine, and serotonin as well as by inhibiting the proliferation of T lymphocytes. Cortisol secretion is also impor-

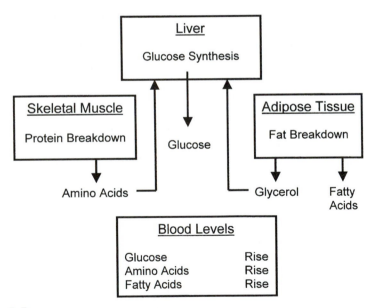

Figure 7–7
Cortisol elevates blood glucose levels by stimulating glucose synthesis in the liver from amino acids and glycerol derived from protein and fat breakdown, respectively.

tant for the normal maintenance of vascular responsiveness to catecholamines by enabling other hormones and neurotransmitters to perform normally. The exact mechanism for this effect is not well understood.

Androgen Action

> Adrenal androgens play an important role in the female but not in the male.

Adrenal androgens do not play a significant role in the male because they do not contribute significantly to testosterone synthesis. The action of testosterone is discussed in the section on male reproductive system in Reproductive Endocrinology.

In the female, adrenal androgens play an important role and are responsible for the development of pubic and axillary hair and for libido (see Reproductive Endocrinology).

Pathology

> • Abnormal adrenocortical secretion can result from alterations in the gland itself, the hypothalamus, or the anterior pituitary.
> • Abnormalities of the adrenal cortex include Addison's disease, Cushing's syndrome, and Conn's syndrome.
> • Abnormalities of the anterior pituitary include Cushing's disease.

Abnormal adrenocortical secretion can result from alterations in the gland itself, the hypothalamus or the anterior pituitary.

Addison's disease usually results from an autoimmune destruction of all three layers of the adrenal cortex. The symptoms parallel the loss of all adrenocortical hormones and include hypoglycemia and weight loss due to the absence of glucocorticoids as well as increased plasma K and hypotension due to the absence of aldosterone. In the absence of adrenocortical hormones there is no negative feedback inhibition of ACTH release, causing blood ACTH levels to be very high. Because MSH is a part of the ACTH molecule, the high levels of ACTH cause skin darkening of patients with Addison's disease.

Cushing's syndrome is excess production of glucocorticoids. Some of the symptoms include hyperglycemia, muscle wasting, obesity, and hypertension. ACTH levels will be low since there is plenty of cortisol to inhibit its release.

Conn's syndrome results from excess aldosterone from an aldosterone-secreting tumor. Symptoms include increased extracellular fluid volume, hypertension, and reduced blood K levels.

Cushing's disease results from oversecretion of ACTH from a pituitary tumor. What distinguishes it from Cushing's syndrome is that the ACTH levels are elevated. All other symptoms are the same.

Adrenal Medulla

> - The adrenal medulla is essentially a neuroendocrine organ that is activated by sympathetic preganglionic nerves.
> - Nerve stimulation results in the release of stored epinephrine and norepinephrine from chromaffin cells.
> - Catecholamines have widespread effects on the cardiovascular system, muscle system, and metabolism.

The adrenal medulla is essentially a modified sympathetic ganglion without post-ganglionic nerves. The secretion of epinephrine and norepinephrine into the blood represents the postganglionic limb. The *chromaffin cells* within the adrenal medulla synthesize epinephrine and norepinephrine from tyrosine and store them within vesicles. More epinephrine than norepinephrine is synthesized (4:1) so when chromaffin cells release their contents, more epinephrine than norepinephrine is secreted.

Catecholamine release occurs during the response to stress. The cardiovascular response to catecholamines is described in chapter 3, Cardiovascular System. The metabolic effect of catecholamines is to prevent a fall in blood glucose levels. The brain senses the blood glucose level and when it falls below the set point, sympathetic preganglionic nerves to the adrenal medulla are activated. These nerves release acetylcholine (ACh), which acts on the muscarinic receptors of chromaffin cells to stimulate an increase in intracellular Ca concentration. The increase in intracellular Ca concentration causes vesicle fusion with the cell membrane and catecholamine release from chromaffin cells.

Catecholamines act on the liver to stimulate glucose synthesis from lactic acid and amino acids. These substrates for glucose synthesis are provided through the action of epinephrine on skeletal muscle and fat cells. In skeletal muscle, epinephrine stimulates glycogen metabolism to lactate, which is released into the blood and used by the liver for glucose synthesis. In adipose cells, epinephrine activates hormone-sensitive lipase causing the breakdown of fats to free fatty acids and glycerol both of which are released into the blood. The liver uses glycerol to make glucose. Finally, catecholamines stimulate glucagon secretion and inhibit insulin release from the pancreas. All these effects are mediated through β-adrenergic G-protein linked membrane receptors.

ENDOCRINE PANCREAS

General Organization

- Cells of the endocrine pancreas are organized into clusters called islets of Langerhans.
- Islets of Langerhans are composed of three cell types—alpha, beta, and delta—that secrete glucagon, insulin, and somatostatin, respectively.
- Blood flow from the beta cells carries insulin past the alpha and delta cells and reduces their secretion of glucagon and somatostatin, respectively.

The cell mass involved in the endocrine function of the pancreas is small (1 to 2%) but the secretions of these cells—insulin, glucagon and somatostatin—have profound effects on the metabolic state of the body. The endocrine pancreas is organized into cell clusters called, *islets of Langerhans*. Each islet is composed of three cell types, *alpha (α), beta (β),* and *delta (δ) cells,* each of which secretes a specific hormone, *insulin, glucagon,* and *somatostatin,* respectively. The secretion of these cells not only acts on tissues of the body but also on other islet cells. Insulin and somatostatin inhibit, while glucagon stimulates, the secretions of other islet cells. The anatomical arrangement of islet cells and their blood supply modulate the effectiveness of these interactions. The β-cells are in the core of the islet and their vasculature supplies the outer cell layer composed of α- and δ-cells. This organization means that insulin is carried immediately past the α- and δ-cells by the blood before reaching and being diluted in the general circulation. Thus the anatomy enhances insulin's inhibitory action. In contrast, glucagon from α-cells reaches the β- and δ-cells only after passing through the systemic circulation. As a consequence, the stimulatory effect of glucagon is delayed because of the time required to sufficiently elevate the blood glucagon concentration.

Insulin

- Insulin is synthesized by β-cells from a prohormone.
- Insulin is the hormone of plenty and is released when metabolic supply (primarily glucose) exceeds the needs of the body.
- Operating through tyrosine kinase receptors on liver, skeletal muscle, and adipose cells, insulin conserves glucose and increases fat storage and protein synthesis.
- Insulin also helps maintain a low blood K ion level by stimulating the Na-K-ATPase pump.

Insulin is synthesized from an 86 amino acid prohormone by enzymatically removing a central amino acid string and linking the remaining strands with two disulfide bonds. The final hormone looks like two railroad tracks (amino acid chains) held together by two ties (disulfide bonds). This synthesis occurs within storage vesicles of the β-cells.

Insulin is released when metabolic supply exceeds metabolic demand. So, in response to a meal, insulin secretion is stimulated. An elevated blood glucose level is the primary stimulus for insulin secretion. Glucose binds to its *glut* 2-transporter on pancreatic β-cells, which carries it into the cell by facilitated transport. Inside the cell, glucose metabolism leads to increased ATP levels, which in turn open K-channels depolarizing the cell and increasing intracellular calcium concentration. Elevated Ca induces fusion of the storage vesicles with the cell membrane and stimulates insulin release. Fatty acids and amino acids also stimulate insulin secretion, presumably through a similar mechanism. Glucagon stimulates insulin secretion by acting directly through a G-protein linked receptor on β-cells as well as indirectly by elevating blood glucose levels (see next section). On the other hand, somatostatin inhibits insulin secretion by acting directly on the β-cells and indirectly by reducing the ability of glucagon to stimulate insulin secretion.

Insulin (see Figure 7–8) reduces blood glucose levels by stimulating glucose uptake into skeletal muscle and fat cells; by stimulating the intracellular conversion of glucose to glycogen in the liver; and by inhibiting the synthesis

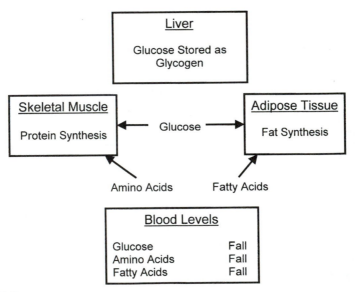

Figure 7–8
Insulin reduces blood glucose levels by stimulating glucose uptake into muscle and fat as well as by inhibiting the formation and release of glucose by the liver.

and subsequence release of new glucose *(gluconeogenesis)* from the liver. Insulin also decreases blood levels of fatty acids and amino acids. Fatty acid levels are decreased because insulin increases fatty acid storage in adipose tissue by inhibiting fatty acid release and breakdown. Blood amino acid levels are reduced by insulin through stimulation of amino acid uptake and protein synthesis in muscle cells. Many of these metabolic effects of insulin are enhanced by insulin inhibition of glucagon secretion. Glucagon opposes the effects of insulin (see next section). This inhibitory effect is facilitated by the anatomical relationship between α- and β-cells as described above.

Insulin also guards against an elevation in blood K ion concentration by increasing tissue K uptake through stimulation of the Na-K-ATPase pump.

Insulin exerts these metabolic effects by stimulating its membrane tyrosine kinase receptor that initiates a signaling cascade leading to protein phosphorylation.

Glucagon

- Glucagon is a single chain of 29 amino acids synthesized by α-cells.
- Glucagon acts primarily on the liver to increase and maintain blood glucose levels.
- Glucagon secretion is increased in response to falling blood glucose and increasing blood amino acid levels.
- Glucagon secretion is inhibited by insulin.
- Glucagon restores blood glucose levels by stimulating glucose synthesis from amino acids and by stimulating fat metabolism.
- Secretion rates of glucagon and insulin change in opposite directions to maintain blood glucose homeostasis.

Glucagon is a single chain of amino acids synthesized by the α-cells. Glucagon's primary function is to prevent a fall in blood glucose levels and together with cortisol, growth hormone, and epinephrine guard against hypoglycemia. Predictably, glucagon is released when blood glucose levels are low, such as during fasting and starvation. However, glucagon secretion is also stimulated by an increase in blood amino acid levels as would occur after a meal. How changes in the levels of these metabolites are sensed and result in changes in glucagon secretion is not clear. Insulin inhibits glucagon secretion by acting directly on α-cells through the insulin-receptor.

To restore blood glucose levels, glucagon (see Figure 7–9) stimulates glucose synthesis by the liver from amino acids and inhibits the ability of the liver to convert glucose to glycogen. In addition, fat metabolism by the liver is increased sparing glucose for tissues that are obligatory glucose users like the central nervous system. Glucagon exerts these effects through its G-protein linked receptor and the subsequent production of the intracellular second messenger, cyclic AMP.

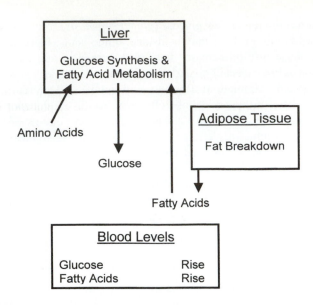

Figure 7–9
Glucagon elevates blood glucose levels by stimulating the synthesis of new glucose by the liver from amino acids. In addition, glucagon stimulates the liver to metabolize fatty acids rather than glucose.

Glucagon and insulin work together to guard against hypoglycemia (glucagon) and hyperglycemia (insulin). Glucagon stimulates breakdown *(catabolism)* of fats and proteins so that fatty acids can be used for fuel and amino acids can be converted to glucose (gluconeogenesis) thereby guarding against a fall in blood glucose levels *(hypoglycemia)*. On the other hand, insulin stimulates glucose uptake from the blood and its conversion to fats and glycogen *(anabolism)* thereby guarding against excess blood glucose *(hyperglycemia)*. To maintain this balance, blood levels of glucagon and insulin exhibit a reciprocal relationship with the blood glucose level determining the balance. In the fed state, insulin levels are high compared to glucagon levels because the high blood glucose stimulates insulin secretion. In addition, the high insulin levels would inhibit glucagon release. However, as blood glucose levels fall during an overnight or a prolonged fast, glucagon secretion increases and insulin secretion decreases so that glucagon levels exceed insulin levels.

Somatostatin

- Somatostatin is a peptide hormone released from δ-cells.
- Somatostatin acts in a paracrine manner to inhibit glucagon and insulin secretion.

Somatostatin is secreted by the δ-cells of the endocrine pancreas. The form secreted by the pancreas is smaller in size than the somatostatin from the GI tract but both have inhibitory action. Pancreatic somatostatin inhibits glucagon and insulin secretion in a paracrine manner, that is, it acts locally rather than being released into the general circulation. Somatostatin secretion is increased in response to a meal and, therefore, acts to modulate the response of insulin and glucagon to a meal.

Diabetes Mellitus

> - Diabetes mellitus is a disease of altered insulin function and is in two forms.
> - Type I is primarily due to the inability of β-cells to produce and secrete insulin; type II is characterized by marked resistance of target tissues to insulin.
> - Metabolic characteristics consist of elevated blood glucose levels, elevated blood amino acid levels, and elevated free fatty acids leading to formation of ketone bodies and acidemia.
> - Blood level of K ions is also elevated.
> - Elevated blood glucose levels lead to osmotic diuresis.
> - Chronic complications of this metabolic disorder affect the eyes, the kidneys, the peripheral nervous system, and the vascular system.

Diabetes mellitus is a disease of altered insulin function resulting either from the loss of insulin production due to destruction of β-cells *(type I)* or resistance of peripheral tissue to insulin *(type II)*. Type I diabetes mellitus usually results from an autoimmune reaction that destroys β-cells. The mechanisms of insulin resistance in type II diabetes mellitus are not understood, but can develop in association with obesity, aging, and various illnesses.

The metabolic response to both forms of diabetes is similar. In the absence of either insulin or its effect, blood glucose levels are high but glucose utilization is low. Glucagon secretion increases because insulin inhibition of its secretion is removed. The absence of effective insulin and the presence of glucagon cause fatty acids to be released, raising their blood levels. Skeletal muscle, liver, and fat cells utilize these fatty acids for energy production and as a result their metabolites, *ketone bodies,* rise in the blood. Ketone bodies are acids and as their blood levels rise, blood pH decreases *(acidemia* due to metabolic acidosis). In addition, plasma K ion levels may be elevated since insulin-induced cellular K uptake is reduced. The elevated plasma K contributes to acidemia by enhancing H ion release from cells. The elevated glucagon-to-insulin ratio also stimulates skeletal muscle protein breakdown to amino acids. The liver inappropriately uses these amino acids to synthesize glucose, which further elevates blood glucose levels. Protein breakdown leads to loss of muscle mass and weakness.

The elevated levels of blood glucose in both forms of diabetes lead to increased urine formation, which can lead to dehydration if water consumption is not increased to match fluid loss. Normally, all filtered glucose is reabsorbed from the tubular fluid by the time it reaches the end of the proximal tubule. But in diabetes mellitus, the high blood glucose level overwhelms the ability of the proximal tubule to reabsorb glucose. This causes glucose to remain in the tubular fluid and appear in the collecting duct. This increases tubular fluid osmolarity retarding water reabsorption by the collecting duct. Urine volume increases, which, if not balanced by increased water consumption, leads to dehydration. Therefore, additional characteristics of diabetes mellitus are polyuria and thirst.

Initially the blood insulin levels of type I and II diabetes mellitus are different. In type I, insulin levels are very low since β-cells cannot synthesize insulin. In type II diabetes, insulin levels are elevated because the high blood glucose stimulates insulin secretion. Over time, "exhaustion" of β-cells due to several mechanisms can lead to reduced insulin secretion, a fall in blood insulin levels, and worsening of the metabolic disorder.

CALCIUM AND PHOSPHATE REGULATION

General Considerations

- Approximately half of the calcium in the blood is ionized, the biologically active form.
- Approximately half of the calcium in the blood is bound to proteins or is complexed with anions such as phosphates and sulfates.
- Blood Ca homeostasis produced through the interaction of bones, kidneys, and small intestine.
- Parathyroid hormone, calcitonin, and vitamin D are the three hormones of Ca homeostasis.
- Hypercalcemia is characterized by constipation, polyuria, and lethargy; hypocalcemia is characterized by spontaneous muscle twitching, cramps, tingling, and numbness.

Only half of the Ca present in the blood is in the ionic form and, therefore, biologically active. The other half is either bound to albumin in the blood or complexed with anions such as phosphate and sulfate.

To maintain a constant blood level, the bones, kidneys, and small intestine interact. For example, in response to a fall in blood Ca levels: (1) *bone resorption* occurs releasing Ca into the blood; (2) the kidney increases Ca reabsorption thereby reducing loss in the urine; and (3) intestinal Ca absorption increases. The coordination of these three tissues is controlled through the actions of parathyroid hormone and vitamin D. Calcitonin affects blood Ca levels but its role is of small physiological significance.

Abnormal blood Ca levels result in symptoms that reflect in part the effect of Ca on nerve excitability. Increased Ca levels *(hypercalcemia)* depress nerve excitability leading to decreased reflex responsiveness, lethargy, coma, and death. In contrast, reduced Ca levels *(hypocalcemia)* lead to increased excitability. This induces spontaneous muscle twitching, cramps, and increased reflex responsiveness.

Parathyroid Gland

> • Parathyroid gland senses blood Ca levels through cell surface receptors.
> • Parathyroid gland secretes PTH in response to reduced blood Ca levels.
> • PTH stimulates bone resorption, renal Ca reabsorption, and intestinal Ca absorption.

There are four parathyroid glands located under the thyroid gland. The cells of the gland have membrane receptors that are sensitive to the ionic Ca concentration of the blood. The receptors are G-protein linked and when stimulated by a fall in blood Ca concentration lead to an increase in intracellular cyclic AMP concentration. Cyclic AMP, through a series of protein phosphorylation reactions, leads to parathyroid hormone (PTH) secretion.

PTH is a small protein (84 amino acids) hormone formed from a preprohormone. The active hormone is stored in vesicles within the parathyroid gland. PTH acts on bone, kidney, and small intestine to return blood Ca to normal levels. The actions of PTH on bone and kidney are mediated through its G-protein linked receptor coupled to cyclic AMP formation and increased protein phosphorylation. The intestinal action of PTH is indirect, mediated through the enhanced renal synthesis of active vitamin D.

PTH enhances bone resorption, that is, dissolution. This is accomplished through the action of PTH on two types of bone cells, *osteoclasts* and *osteoblasts*. PTH stimulates osteoclasts to remove calcium from the bone matrix and inhibits osteoblasts from making new bone. The result is the release of both Ca and phosphate from bone. If PTH had no other effects, this would not raise the ionic Ca concentration of the blood because calcium phosphate complexes would form. However, PTH also acts on the kidney where it has two effects: increased phosphate excretion and increased Ca reabsorption. PTH inhibits renal proximal tubule phosphate reabsorption by decreasing the transport maximum of the Na-phosphate uptake carrier. Because of this effect, the carrier becomes saturated at lower filtered loads enabling more phosphate to escape reabsorption and to be excreted *(phosphaturia)*. The increased phosphate excretion eliminates the phosphate released from bone enabling the free ionic Ca concentration in the blood to rise. PTH fur-

ther elevates blood Ca levels by acting on the distal renal tubule to stimulate Ca reabsorption. Finally, PTH acts on the kidney to stimulate renal 1α-hydroxylase, the
enzyme that converts the inactive to the active form of vitamin D. The active form
of vitamin D acts on the small intestine to increase Ca absorption.

Vitamin D

- Vitamin D (cholecalciferol) is a steroid obtained from the diet or synthe-
  sized by the skin.
- Active form of vitamin D (1,25 dihydroxycholecalciferol) is formed in
  the kidneys through the action of 1α-hydroxylase.
- Activity of 1α-hydroxylase is influenced by the blood levels of Ca and
  PTH.
- Vitamin D elevates blood levels of both Ca and phosphate through ac-
  tions on the small intestines, kidneys, and bone.

Vitamin D or *cholecalciferol* is a steroid that is either obtained in the diet or synthesized by the skin from cholesterol through the effect of ultraviolet light. It has
no physiological action. In the liver it is converted to *25-hydroxycholecalciferol*,
which is also without biological activity. The kidney contains *1α-hydroxylase*
that hydroxylates 25-hydroxycholecalciferol to *1,25-dihydroxycholecalciferol*,
the active hormone (1,25-vitamin D). Decreased blood levels of Ca or increased
levels of PTH stimulate the activity of 1α-hydroxylase and increase the formation of 1,25-vitamin D.

1,25-vitamin D acts on the small intestine, kidneys, and bone to elevate
blood levels of both Ca and phosphate. As a steroid hormone, its mechanism of
action is to induce protein synthesis through increased DNA transcription. In the
intestine, 1,25-vitamin D stimulates the synthesis of an intracellular Ca-binding
protein, *calbindin*. Calbindin binds four Ca ions and in some yet to be determined way, enhances Ca absorption. In the kidney, 1,25-vitamin D stimulates reabsorption of both Ca and phosphate. This is in contrast to the action of PTH,
which had opposite effects on renal Ca and phosphate reabsorption. In bone,
1,25-vitamin D stimulates osteoclast activity, the resorption of bone and the release of Ca and phosphate into the blood.

Calcitonin

- Calcitonin is synthesized by parafollicular cells or C cells of the thyroid
  gland.
- Increased blood Ca levels stimulate calcitonin secretion.   *(continued)*

> (*continued*)
> • Calitonin inhibits osteoclast bone resorption reducing blood Ca levels.
> • Its physiological function is not well defined.

Calcitonin is a small protein (32 amino acids) hormone produced by *parafollicular cells* or *C cells* of the thyroid gland. The C cells are separate from the follicular cells responsible for thyroid hormone synthesis. The primary stimulus for calcitonin secretion is elevated blood Ca levels. Calcitonin inhibits osteoclast-induced bone resorption thereby decreasing Ca release and enabling Ca levels to fall through normal renal excretion. Calcitonin does not seem to participate in moment-to-moment regulation of blood Ca levels and its physiological role is not clear at this time.

REPRODUCTIVE ENDOCRINOLOGY

Sexual Differentiation

> • Sexual differentiation is determined at three levels: chromosomes, gonads, and phenotype.
> • Males have XY and females have XX chromosomes.
> • Female characteristics develop spontaneously in the absence of the Y chromosome.
> • Y chromosome contains the gene—sex-determining region (SRY)—that is necessary for the development of male characteristics.
> • Gonads are composed of three cell types in both males and females: supporting cells (Sertoli or granulosa cells); stromal cells (Leydig or theca cells); and germ cells (spermatogonia or oocytes).
> • Fetal testes secrete two hormones—antimullerian hormone and testosterone—that are essential for development of the male gonads and internal genitalia; in their absence female gonads and internal genitalia develop.
> • Dihydrotestosterone is responsible for development of male external genitalia.

Sexual differentiation begins with the establishment of chromosomal sex, which directs gonadal sex, and leads to development of secondary sex characteristics that define the male or female phenotype. In most cases the chromosomal sex of the fetus results in a specific phenotype. However, ambiguities exist where the phenotype is inconsistent with the chromosomal or gonadal sex of the individual because of inappropriate hormone release or function.

At the chromosome level, maleness is defined by the presence of XY chromosomes, and femaleness is defined by the presence of XX chromosomes. The Y chromosome contains a gene, *SRY (sex-determining region, Y chromosome)* that encodes a regulator of DNA transcription, which initiates a cascade of events resulting in testicular development. The SRY gene is necessary but not sufficient for the development of maleness because hormones (androgens) from the testes are also necessary along with androgen receptors on target tissues.

Gonads are composed of hormone-producing and germ cells. Prior to the first 7 to 8 weeks in the developing fetus, gonads and internal genitalia are identical in both sexes. The gonads consist of supporting cells [Sertoli (in males) or granulose cells (in females)], stromal cells [Leydig (males) or theca cells (females)] and germ cells [spermatogonia (males) or oocytes (female)]. The internal genitalia of the early fetus consist of a dual ductal system composed of *wolffian* and *mullerian ducts*. If the SRY gene is present (Y chromosome), at approximately 8 weeks the gonads begin to differentiate into the testis and secrete two essential hormones: *antimullerian hormone (AMH)* from the *Sertoli cells* and *testosterone* from the *Leydig cells*. AMH, a member of the TGH-β family of growth factors, inhibits the development of the mullerian duct, which would have become the female genital tract. Testosterone stimulates development of the wolffian duct, which gives rise to the epididymis, the vas deferens, the seminal vesicles, and the ejaculatory ducts. In the absence of the SRY gene, the gonads differentiate into ovaries and the mullerian ducts develop into the fallopian tubes, the body and cervix of the uterus, and the upper third of the vagina. At the same time, the wolffian ducts degenerate. Fetal ovaries, unlike fetal testes, do not secrete significant levels of hormone so the development of ovaries and the internal genitalia occur spontaneously in the absence of inhibitory factors (eg, AMH).

Just like the development of the gonads and internal genitalia, development of female-specific external genitalia—the lower third of the vagina and the labia—occurs unless opposed by hormone action. Development of male external genitalia—the penis and scrotum—and prostate gland begins around the 10th week and requires the hormone, *dihydrotestosterone*. Testosterone, released from Leydig cells, is converted to dihydrotestosterone by the enzyme, *5α-reductase,* located on the surface of target tissue. Dihydrotestosterone causes differentiation of the penis and formation of the scrotum as well as inhibition of the development of female external genitalia.

The specific roles of testosterone and dihydrotestosterone in male sexual differentiation can be seen from cases where the action of one of the hormones is absent. If 5α-reductase is absent or its receptor does not function, testes and male internal genitalia develop (supported by testosterone) but external male genitalia are absent (supported by dihydrotestosterone). Such an individual would have a female phenotype but be male based on chromosomal and gonadal characteristics.

Puberty

> - Onset of puberty is marked by pulsatile secretion of GnRH, FSH, and LH.
> - In the male, FSH stimulates sperm and Sertoli cell development while LH stimulates Leydig cell proliferation and testosterone secretion.
> - In the female, FSH stimulates follicle development and, along with LH, the synthesis of estradiol.
> - Testosterone and estradiol stimulate the development of secondary sex characteristics and a growth spurt in the male and female, respectively.

The pulsatile secretion of GnRH from the hypothalamus with the subsequent pulsatile secretion of FSH and LH from the anterior pituitary marks the onset of puberty. In females the transition to puberty begins around the age of 6 to 8 years and in males between 9 and 10 years. The mechanism responsible for the onset of pulsatile GnRH release is not known but may involve changes in the neural input to the hypothalamic cells that release GnRH as well as a change in the ability of these cells to synthesize and secrete GnRH. In addition, the sensitivity of anterior pituitary cells to GnRH increases, enhancing the secretion of FSH and LH.

In the male, pulsatile levels of FSH stimulate development of seminiferous tubules, sperm, and Sertoli cells, which results in enlargement of the testes. The pulsatile levels of LH stimulate Leydig cell proliferation and testosterone secretion. The elevated levels of testosterone are responsible for the development of secondary sex characteristics that include increase in penis size, darkening of the color of the scrotum, growth of axillary hair, male hair pattern, lowering of the voice, and development of sebaceous glands. In addition, testosterone stimulates linear growth and skeletal muscle hypertrophy as well as closure of the long bone epiphyses, ultimately limiting growth. Some of these responses result directly from the action of testosterone and some from the action of dihydrotestosterone produced locally by the target tissue.

In the female, pulsatile levels of FSH stimulate the development of the follicle and along with LH stimulate estradiol synthesis and secretion from the ovaries. Estradiol stimulates development of the breasts and reproductive organs. In addition, it is responsible for the growth and development of the uterus, fallopian tubes, cervix, and vagina. The pulsatile swings in estradiol increase in magnitude as puberty progresses. Each of these increasing swings causes a parallel swing in the magnitude of uterine endometrium development. At some point, sufficient endometrial development occurs with each cycle that as estradiol levels fall, the first menstruation occurs. On average, the onset of the menstrual cycle *(menarche)* occurs at 12 years of age. The appearance and distribution of pubic and axillary hair is stimulated by testosterone as in the male. However, testosterone is produced locally from *androstenedione* released from the adrenal cortex and ovaries. Androstenedione is converted to testosterone by hair follicle cells. Therefore, a normally functioning adrenal cortex is essential in the female for normal pubic and axillary hair growth. The increasing release of androstenedione from the adrenal cortex, called *adrenarche*, is independent of the pulsatile changes in GnRH-FSH-LH, begins at about 7 to 8 years of age and peaks at 13 to 15 years of age.

Male Reproductive System

- Testes are composed of seminiferous tubules that produce sperm and Leydig cells, which produce testosterone.
- Spermatogenesis results from conversion of spermatogonia to mature sperm through mitosis, meiosis, and differentiation.
- Sertoli cells of the seminiferous tubules support sperm development as well as surround and isolate developing sperm from the blood supply.
- Leydig cells, under the influence of LH, secrete testosterone.
- FSH and testosterone acting through Sertoli cells enable spermatogenesis.
- Blood levels of testosterone and inhibin feed back to regulate pituitary release of FSH and LH.

The testes are composed of a network of tubules *(seminiferous tubules)* designed for the production and transport of sperm and interstitial cells *(Leydig cells)* designed for the synthesis of testosterone. Seminiferous tubules make up approximately 80% of the testes and are organized into densely packed lobules. Between these lobules is a compact material composed of connective tissue, Leydig cells, and smooth muscle cells. The testes are normally located outside the body cavity in the scrotum because sperm production is optimal at a temperature that is 1 to 2 degrees cooler than core body temperature.

Seminiferous tubules are lined with a basement membrane on which sit specialized epithelial cells, the *Sertoli cells* (see Figure 7–10). The Sertoli cells are tall columnar cells that extend from the basement membrane into the lumen of the tubule. Between the Sertoli cells and also sitting on the basement membrane are immature germ cells called *spermatogonia*. Above the spermatogonia are tight junctions connecting adjacent Sertoli cells. These tight junctions limit the movement of material from the interstitium into the lumen of the seminiferous tubules and form the *blood-testes barrier*. This barrier has several consequences. First, it separates the spermatogonia from the lumen. Before spermatogonia become mature, sperm must pass through the tight junctions. Therefore mature

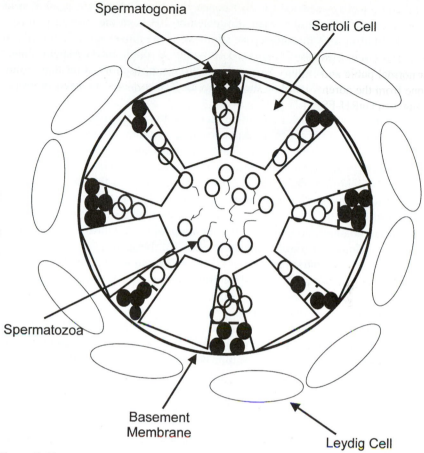

Figure 7–10

The testes are composed of maturing sperm (spermatogonia, spermatozoa), Sertoli cells, and Leydig cells that interact to ensure a continuous production of sperm.

sperm are outside of the blood-testes barrier and are not recognized as "self" by the body's immune system. Consequently, males can become immunized against their own sperm. The blood-testes barrier also separates maturing sperm from the nutrients in the blood. So one of the functions of the Sertoli cells is to provide these nutrients. Sertoli cells also serve a phagocytic function, digesting damaged germ cells. In addition, they assist in the detachment of sperm into the lumen.

The seminiferous tubules collect into a network of ducts that eventually lead to a single duct, the *epididymis*. The epididymis is the primary site for maturation and storage of sperm. Sexual arousal stimulates contraction of smooth muscle cells lining the epididymis, propelling the sperm into the *vas deferens* and the urethra.

Leydig cells, scattered in the connective tissue between seminiferous tubules, secrete testosterone when stimulated by LH from the anterior pituitary. The rate-limiting step in testosterone synthesis is the movement of intracellular cholesterol into the mitochondria. LH acting through its G-protein linked membrane receptor initiates a cascade of protein phosphorylation that stimulates this movement as well as the activity of key enzymes involved in testosterone synthesis.

Spermatogenesis consists of three phases: mitosis, meiosis, and differentiation or *spermiogenesis*. It begins at puberty and continues until senescence. One full cycle of spermatogenesis requires about 65 days and begins with a spermatogonium undergoing 4 mitotic divisions to produce 16 *primary spermatocytes* each with 46 chromosomes. These cells move away from the basement membrane through the tight junction between Sertoli cells. Next, 2 meiotic divisions occur resulting in 64 cells called *spermatids*, each with 23 chromosomes. Spermatid differentiation into mature sperm, or *spermiogenesis,* involves reorganization of the cell nucleus toward the putative head of the sperm, loss of most of the cytoplasm, and concentration of the mitochondria around the base of the flagella and elongation of the flagellum. Maturation continues as the sperm *(spermatozoa)* passes through the epididymis to the ejaculatory duct.

Spermatogenesis requires FSH from the anterior pituitary, testosterone from Leydig cells, and normal Sertoli cell function. FSH release is under the control of GnRH from the hypothalamus. Testosterone release from Leydig cells is controlled by LH, which in turn is controlled by GnRH. Both FSH and testosterone exert their effects through the Sertoli cells, which is why normal Sertoli cell function is critical. FSH through its G-protein linked receptors stimulates Sertoli cells to make *androgen-binding protein (ABP)*. ABP binds testosterone released from Leydig cells, increasing the local testosterone concentration around Sertoli cells thereby increasing the effectiveness of testosterone. FSH has other effects on Sertoli cells that are not clearly defined but are necessary for normal Sertoli cell function. Testosterone acting through intracellular receptors induces the expression by Sertoli cells of specific proteins essential for sperm development.

FSH, LH and testosterone levels are regulated through the release of GnRH, negative feedback by testosterone, and production of an inhibitor. In the adult male, GnRH secretion is pulsatile with a frequency of 8 to 14 cycles per day. This results in cyclical changes in FSH, LH, and testosterone secretion. The origin of the pulsatile GnRH secretion is unknown, but its frequency and effectiveness is modulated in two ways. One way is through testosterone. Elevation in blood testosterone levels feed back on the anterior pituitary to inhibit LH secretion as well as on the hypothalamus to inhibit GnRH secretion. The second way is through a secretion from Sertoli cells. Elevated blood levels of FSH stimulate Sertoli cells to secrete a protein called *inhibin*. Inhibin acts on the anterior pituitary where it reduces the ability of GnRH to stimulate FSH release.

Female Reproductive System

- Ovary has three regions: cortex composed of follicles; medulla composed of stromal and hormone-producing cells; and hilum, the point of entry of blood vessels and nerves.
- Follicles are composed of three cell types: oocytes, granulosa, thecal.
- Initial development of oocytes begins in fetal life, but maturation is delayed until puberty when single oocytes mature and are released monthly for the next 4 decades.
- Progesterone and estradiol are main steroid hormones produced by the ovaries—estradiol from granulosa cells and progesterone from many cell types.
- Estradiol is released prior to ovulation, progesterone after ovulation; both prepare the uterus for egg implantation.
- FSH stimulates monthly development of follicles, LH stimulates monthly ovulation, and both stimulate synthesis and secretion of progesterone and estradiol.
- Corpus luteum, the postovulation follicle, secretes estradiol and progesterone to sustain the egg and uterus if fertilization and implantation occur.

The ovary is organized into three layers. The outer cortex contains the follicles composed of oocytes, granulosa, and thecal cells. The medullary layer is composed of a variety of cells and connective material. The innermost layer is the hilum, which is the entry point for blood vessels and nerves.

Oocytes and spermatozoa share some characteristics but also have many differences. Both have similar embryonic origins, require supporting cells (granulosa and Sertoli cells), are stimulated by FSH and LH, depend upon steroid hormones, and are the only cells of the body that undergo meiosis. However, they also differ in many ways. The oocytes, being the largest cells of the body, are much bigger than the sperm, which are structured more for mobility. Oocytes are released into the peritoneal cavity; sperm are formed and released into a tubular system. Even though both cells undergo meiosis, oocytes undergo the first meiosis during fetal development and do not complete the second until some time between puberty and the next 40 years. In spermatozoa, meiosis begins at puberty, is completed within 65 days, and is repeated by other spermatozoa continuously until senescence.

The formation of the functional unit of the ovary—ovarian follicle with a single enclosed oocyte—begins in the fetus but is delayed and not completed until after puberty. Development of the oocyte and the granulosa and thecal cells of the follicle occur in parallel. During early fetal life, germ cells divide repeatedly forming approximately 7 million *oogonia*. Each oogonium begins but does not complete the first or prophase of meiosis and becomes a *primary oocyte*. Between birth and puberty most of the primary oocytes are lost so that approximately 400,000 remain at the beginning of puberty. While the primary oocyte develops, granulosa cells proliferate and sustain the oocyte by providing nutrients and steroid hormones. The primary oocyte and the surrounding layer of granulosa cells are called a *primary follicle*. The primary follicle and oocyte do not undergo further changes until after puberty and the beginning of menses.

With each menstrual cycle a small number of primary follicles (6–10) begins to mature with only a single primary follicle completing the cycle to ovulation. It is not known what causes a specific collection of follicles to begin this process, but it is characterized by increased granulosa and theca cell growth, increased estradiol production by granulosa cells, and by accumulation of FSH within the lumen of the follicle. Because of these changes, the primary follicle increases in size from less than 1 mm in diameter to over 20 mm. This final structure is called a *graafian follicle* and only one primary follicle reaches this stage. By some unknown mechanism, around day 5 to 7 of the menstrual cycle the progression of other primary follicles is suppressed and a single graafian follicle becomes the *dominant follicle*. The dominant follicle enlarges, and on the 15th day of the menstruation cycle, it ruptures releasing the oocyte *(ovulation)*. As described below, ovulation is initiated by a surge in blood LH levels, which also induces the primary oocyte to complete the first meiotic division and to begin the second a few hours before ovulation. The released oocyte is called a *secondary oocyte,* and if fertilized, rapidly completes the second meiotic division.

The menstrual cycle is divided into three phases: follicular, ovulation, and luteal. Movement through these phases occurs because of the coordinated actions of FSH, LH, estradiol, and progesterone. The follicular phase begins at the end of the previous menstrual cycle and lasts for 15 days. This is the phase during which a small group of primary follicles undergoes the transformations leading to the generation of a single dominant follicle. During the first half of the follicular phase, FSH levels are elevated and stimulate the transition from primary to dominant follicle. FSH stimulates granulosa cell proliferation and their secretion of estradiol. Estradiol acts on the uterus to stimulate endometrium development and vascularization in preparation for implantation of the fertilized egg. By mid-follicular phase, FSH levels begin to decline because the rising levels of estradiol feed back negatively on the anterior pituitary reducing secretion. However, FSH has induced an increase in the number of its own receptors on granulosa cells. This means that even though blood FSH levels are declining, effective stimulation of estradiol secretion occurs. LH levels slowly increase during this time also and stimulate estradiol secretion by granulosa cells and androgens by thecal cells. Androgens (androstenedione and testosterone) are converted to estradiol by granulosa cells (see description below) as well as help to suppress maturation of all but the dominant follicle. The combined effects of FSH and LH on granulosa cells cause blood estradiol levels to rise rapidly near the end of the follicular phase. The high estradiol levels now exert a positive feedback effect on FSH and LH secretion, which results in a dramatic surge in FSH and LH levels.

This surge in gonadotropin release signals the end of the follicular phase and the beginning of ovulation. The high LH level, causes the dominant follicle to rupture and the release of the oocyte. Immediately after ovulation, FSH and LH levels fall precipitously. The granulosa and theca cells of the ruptured follicle reorganize and form the *corpus luteum*. This begins the luteal phase of the menstrual cycle, which lasts about 14 days. LH is important in maintaining the structural and functional integrity of the corpus luteum. In addition, LH stimulates the corpus luteum to secrete progesterone and estradiol. Both hormones act on the uterus to continue its preparation for implantation that was begun by estradiol during the follicular phase. Progesterone levels exceed those of estradiol during the luteal phase and increase the secretory activity and vascularity of the uterus.

In the absence of implantation, the corpus luteum degenerates, progesterone and estradiol levels fall, and the endometrium is lost (menses). However, if implantation occurs, degeneration of the corpus luteum is prevented (see below) and it plays a critical role in sustaining the developing embryo until the placenta takes its place.

Granulosa and theca cells interact during the menstrual cycle to ensure adequate secretion of steroid hormones (see Figure 7–11). Granulosa cells are deficient in the enzyme 17,20-lyase, (P450c17) and so cannot convert progesterone to androstenedione, a key intermediate needed for estradiol synthesis. Theca cells contain 17,20-lyase and so can synthesize androstenedione and testosterone but not the aromatase enzyme (P450arom) needed to carry the synthesis through to estradiol. To enable granulosa cells to synthesize estradiol in the absence of the key enzyme, theca cells provide granulosa cells with the needed substrates, androstenedione and testosterone. In this way, the step between progesterone and androstenedione is bypassed. The granulosa cells contain aromatase and the other necessary enzymes to convert these substrates to estradiol. Because of this interdependence between granulosa and theca cells, estradiol secretion depends upon stimulation by both LH and FSH. LH stimulates theca cell production of androstenedione and testosterone, which diffuse to the granulosa cells where they are converted to estradiol by FSH stimulation of aromatase.

Pregnancy

- Fertilization of the oocyte occurs within 24 hours of ovulation in the distal end of the oviduct.
- Fertilized egg completes second meiosis and divides repeatedly to form multicelled blastocyst.

(continued)

(*continued*)
- Blastocyst implants in uterine wall within 5 days of ovulation.
- After implantation, blastocyst secretes human chorionic gonadotropin (hCG), which signals the corpus luteum to continue secreting progesterone and estradiol.
- Progesterone is produced from cholesterol by the placenta and estriol through the interaction of the placenta and fetal adrenal cortex and liver.
- Progesterone and estriol support development of the fetus as well as maternal breast development.
- The mechanism by which parturition is initiated is unclear but involves an interplay between progesterone, prostaglandins, and oxytocin that increases the frequency of uterine contraction.

The released oocyte is swept into the oviduct where it becomes fertilized within 24 hours. Upon sperm penetration, the oocyte completes the second meiotic divi-

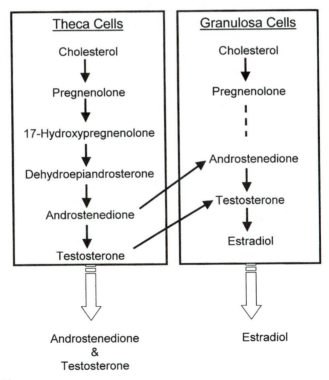

Figure 7–11
The theca and granulose cells of the ovary interact to ensure adequate production of androgens (androstenedione, testosterone) and estradiol.

sion and then after fertilization, it divides rapidly forming a *blastocyst*. Within 5 days the blastocyst traverses the oviduct and implants in the endometrium. The high progesterone levels produced by the corpus luteum are essential for implantation. The outer cellular layer of the blastocyst, called the *trophoblast*, forms the fetal portion of the placenta and begins to secrete *human chorionic gonadotropin (hCG)*. hCG signals the corpus luteum that implantation has occurred. hCG prevents the corpus luteum from degenerating and stimulates it to continue to secrete progesterone and estradiol. hCG is detectable in the urine within 9 days of ovulation and is the basis of the pregnancy test.

During the first 13 weeks of pregnancy (first trimester), the corpus luteum is responsible for progesterone and estrogen secretion after which time the placenta assumes this responsibility. The placenta synthesizes progesterone from cholesterol removed from the maternal blood. However, the synthesis of estriol, the major form of estrogen during pregnancy, requires an interaction between the mother, the placenta, and the fetus (see Figure 7–12). First the placenta takes up cholesterol from the mother's blood and converts it to pregnenolone because it lacks 17 α-hydroxylase and cannot carry the synthesis further. Pregnenolone passes into the fetal circulation where it is first converted to dehydroepinandros-terone-sulfate (DHEA-sulfate) by the fetal adrenal and then to 16-OH DHEA-sulfate by the fetal liver. 16-OH DHEA-sulfate passes back to the placenta, which is capable of converting this substrate to estriol through the action of the aromatase enzyme. All during fetal development, progesterone and estriol levels in maternal and fetal blood continue to rise.

After approximately 40 weeks, parturition is signaled. One stimulus is the size of the fetus, which distends the uterus initiating contractions. However, the final signal for coordinated contractions and expulsion of the fetus is not clear. It

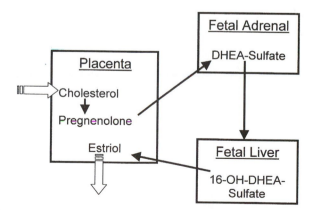

Figure 7–12
Ensuring an adequate production of estriol during pregnancy requires exchange of substances between the maternal blood, the placenta, the fetal adrenal gland, and the fetal liver.

seems to involve interplay between progesterone, prostaglandins (PGE_2 and PGF_2-α), and oxytocin.

In addition to supporting fetal development, progesterone and estrogen stimulate the development and growth of the maternal breasts. Estrogen also stimulates prolactin secretion by the anterior pituitary, which participates in breast development. At parturition, levels of all three hormones fall, but the breasts are ready for milk production and release induced by increased prolactin and oxytocin levels brought on by suckling.

· C H A P T E R · 8 ·

TEMPERATURE REGULATION

·

BASIC PRINCIPLES AND ORGANIZATION
Physics of Heat Transfer

- Heat transfer occurs by radiation, conduction, convection, evaporation.
- Body makes use of all four to maintain temperature.

Heat is transferred by radiation, conduction, convection, and evaporation. *Radiation* is heat movement in the form of infrared heat rays. The body gives off infrared heat if it is warmer than the surrounding environment and absorbs infrared heat if it is cooler than the surrounding environment. Radiation can dissipate up to 15% of the heat generated by the body if surrounding conditions are appropriate.

Conduction is the transfer of heat between two surfaces that are in direct physical contact. Even though our bodies make contact with a variety of surfaces, like the seat of a chair, this does not represent a significant form of conductive heat loss. However, conductive heat transfer between the body and the surrounding air is significant. Usually the surrounding air is cooler than the body, so conduction of heat to the air represents an important way for the body to dissipate heat (approximately 15%). A limitation of conduction is that as heat is transferred, a layer of air close to the surface of the body is warmed to body temperature. This reduces conduction, because the two surfaces (body and air) are now at the same temperature. When the body is immersed in water, conduction between the body and the water occurs. However, in contrast to air, the ability of water to absorb heat without changing temperature is much greater. This means that the body cannot warm the layer of water near the surface of the body significantly and so water removes heat from the body more effectively than air.

Convection transfers heat by physically refreshing the surfaces that are conducting heat. As was discussed above, conduction between the body and air is self-limiting because the body warms the layer of air next to the body. However, if the air is continuously replaced with cooler air, as when there is a breeze (convection), conduction continues. Therefore, convection enhances conduction. In our daily lives, the effect of convection is reflected in the magnitude of the "wind-chill factor" reported by weather forecasters. Approximately 15% of heat generated by the body can be dissipated in this way.

The *evaporation* of water from the surface of the body removes heat from the body because the heat needed to change water from a liquid to a gas is derived from the heat of the body. Evaporation of sweat from the surface of the body is the most significant mechanism that the body has for dissipating heat.

Sensing Body Temperature

- Core body temperature is a controlled variable.
- Heat is generated by metabolism primarily in the brain, heart, liver, and skeletal muscle.
- Anterior hypothalamus is the integration center for temperature control.
- Anterior hypothalamus and skin sense body temperature.
- Fever alters the temperature set point of the hypothalamus.

The *core body temperature,* that is, the temperature of the interior of the body, is a controlled variable that is maintained within narrow limits. Normal cellular metabolism, primarily by the brain, heart, liver and skeletal muscle, generates heat. Therefore, in response to changes in metabolic activity and/or environmental conditions, the core body temperature can change. Optimal enzyme activity occurs at a specific temperature (approximately 98°F or 37°C) and so, the body must dissipate or conserve heat to maintain a constant core temperature. Core body temperature is difficult to measure in a noninvasive manner, so it is estimated from oral and rectal temperatures.

The anterior hypothalamus is a temperature sensor as well as the integration center controlling effector systems involved in regulating core temperature. Temperature sensors are also located on the skin and are bare nerve endings. They can be divided into two groups based on their response to temperature. One group is most active at high temperatures and the other group is most active at low temperatures. These nerve endings send their information to the anterior hypothalamus.

The temperature set point of the hypothalamus is raised when *fever* occurs. In response to infection, the body produces *interleukin-1,* which acts on the anterior hypothalamus to raise the temperature set point initiating reflexes to elevate body temperature. This effect of interleukin-1 is mediated in part through stimulating the production of prostaglandin E_2 (PGE_2). Aspirin reduces fever by inhibiting cyclooxygenase, the enzyme responsible for PGE_2 formation, thereby preventing the change in the temperature set point.

Sweat Glands

- Sweat glands consist of secretory cells and ductule cells.
- Secretory cells produce an isotonic salt solution the composition of which is altered as it flows past the ductule cells.
- Sympathetic-cholinergic nerves increase rate of sweat formation.
- Maximum secretory ability changes with acclimatization.

Sweat glands are structurally similar to salivary and pancreatic secretory glands in that they consist of secretory and ductule cells. Secretory cells form a coiled tubular structure that lies in the subdermal layer of the skin. They secrete a salt solution that is essentially isotonic to blood. It contains no protein and so is an ultrafiltrate of the blood (similar to the glomerular filtrate). Sodium and chloride ions are the major ionic constituents of the secretion. The ductule cells form a long tube through which the fluid reaches the surface of the skin. As the fluid moves through the duct, sodium ions are removed and water follows. This concentrates the sweat. The extent of this concentration depends upon the rate of sweat formation. The slower the rate, the more concentration occurs and the lower the sodium content.

Sympathetic-cholinergic nerves innervate sweat glands and when nerve activity increases, the rate of sweat formation increases. Sympathetic-cholinergic nerves are anatomically sympathetic, that is, they have a short preganglionic nerve fiber and a long postganglionic nerve fiber, but the postganglionic nerve fiber releases acetylcholine rather than norepinephrine. Muscarinic receptors on the secretory cells are stimulated by the acetylcholine and increase their rate of sweat formation.

The production rate and composition of sweat changes when one acclimatizes to a hot environment. Acclimatization takes up to 6 weeks to occur and results in two changes. The first is that the maximum volume of sweat generated can double or triple from 1 L/hour to 2 to 3 L/hour. Secondly, the Na content is lower. At high secretory rates one would expect that the Na content of the sweat would be high because the ductule cells would not be able to remove the Na ions. However, with acclimatization the amount of aldosterone secreted from the adrenal cortex increases, which stimulates Na reabsorption by the ductule cells. This reduces the sodium lost in sweat. The elevated aldosterone levels result directly from the fall in extracellular sodium chloride produced by sweating. An unacclimatized person sweating at the maximum rate will lose 15 to 30 g of salt a day, but this is reduced to 3 to 5 g per day after acclimatization.

REFLEX COMPENSATION FOR BODY TEMPERATURE CHANGES

Reflex Response to Cold

- Objective of body is to reduce heat loss and increase heat production.
- Reducing heat loss occurs by decreasing skin blood flow and through behavioral responses.
- Increasing heat production occurs through metabolic effects of thyroxin and catecholamines as well as by shivering.
- Sustained exposure to extreme cold depresses hypothalamic temperature control mechanisms and produces dilation of skin vasculature.

When a fall in core body temperature is detected by the hypothalamus, the reflex compensation involves reducing heat loss and generating more heat by increasing metabolic rate and through shivering.

Heat loss is reduced by decreasing skin blood flow. The anterior hypothalamus activates nerve cells in the posterior hypothalamus, which in turn activate sympathetic nerves to skin blood vessels causing vasoconstriction. This reduced blood flow decreases heat loss by radiation, conduction, convection, and evaporation. In addition, behavioral responses occur that can include: (1) a desire to move into a warmer environment; (2) increasing the amount of clothing worn; and (3) assuming a body posture that reduces heat loss.

One way to increase heat production is to stimulate metabolism, that is, *chemical thermogenesis*. The anterior hypothalamus initiates thyroxin release through the TRF–TSH–T_3 axis. Thyroxin stimulates cellular metabolism and thereby raises heat production. Catecholamines released either from sympathetic nerve endings or from the adrenal medulla act on fat cells (primarily brown fat) to decrease the efficiency with which their mitochondria transfer energy to ATP during oxidative phosphorylation. Because of this decrease in efficiency heat is released. Chemical thermogenesis in humans is small but can increase heat production 10 to 15%.

Another way to increase heat production is through shivering. The posterior hypothalamus contains an area called the *primary motor center for shivering*. This area is normally inhibited by the temperature center in the anterior hypothalamus but when core temperature falls, this inhibition is removed. Nerves from the shivering center activate motor nerves to skeletal muscles and stretch receptors located there. This increase in motor nerve activity initiates the burst of muscle contractions characteristic of shivering.

Reflex Response to Heat

- Objective of the body is to increase heat loss and to reduce excess heat generation.
- An increase in heat loss occurs by increasing skin blood flow and by increasing sweat formation.
- Heat generation is reduced by inhibition of chemical thermogenesis and shivering.
- Sustained maximum heat dissipation leads to heat exhaustion followed by heat stroke because of cardiovascular collapse.

When core temperature increases, the body initiates reflexes to increase heat loss and to reduce excess heat generation.

Heat loss is increased by increasing skin blood flow and the rate of sweat formation. Skin blood flow is increased by two different mechanisms both involving sympathetic nerves. One way that the body uses to increase skin blood flow is to decrease sympathetic adrenergic nerve stimulation of skin arteriolar smooth muscle causing vasodilation. The second way involves an increase (not a decrease) in the activity of sympathetic nerve activity that produces vasodilation. How the increase in sympathetic nerve activity accomplishes vasodilation is not known, but it may involve the release of vasodilator substances possibly from the sweat glands that are stimulated by the sympathetic nerves. The increase in skin blood flow can increase heat loss by as much as eight times through radiation and conduction.

Heat loss can also be increased through an increase in sweat formation, which increases evaporative loss. Increased sympathetic nerve activity to sweat glands stimulates the rate of sweat production. This is the most effective mechanism that the body has to remove heat from the body, therefore anything that limits this mechanism will greatly reduce the ability of an individual to function in a hot environment (see below).

The body also reduces the generation of excess heat. The shivering center is inhibited and stimuli that would initiate chemical thermogenesis are reduced. Also, behavioral adaptation occurs including a decrease in physical activity, movement to cool locations, and increasing heat loss through convection by mechanically moving the air surrounding the body.

Sustained maximum heat dissipation can lead to cardiovascular collapse. Continued sweating at high rates (2–3 L/hr) reduces extracellular fluid volume and salt content. The loss of extracellular volume compromises the ability of the cardiovascular system to meet the metabolic and temperature control needs of the body. The normal reflex response to a fall in blood volume (extracellular volume) includes a reduction in skin blood flow (compromises heat dissipation), so available volume is used to perfuse the brain and heart. Reflexes to dissipate heat normally include an increase in skin blood flow, which reduces the blood available to perfuse essential organs. The body must "decide" which of these two reflex compensations dominates. In the end, thermal regulation dominates causing the blood pressure to fall as the blood is directed toward the skin. As a consequence, the person faints. This is called *heat exhaustion* or *heat syncope*. When this occurs, core body temperature is not substantially elevated because sweating is occurring so the skin is moist. However, if body temperature rises to the point that tissue damage occurs, the body's ability to lower temperature will be compromised and core temperature will rise. This is called *heat stroke* and is a severe medical condition that requires immediate lowering of the body temperature to prevent further damage and death.